Management of Acute Coronary Syndromes

Management of Acute Coronary Syndromes

Eli V. Gelfand

*Director of Ambulatory Cardiology, Beth Israel
Deaconess Medical Center, Harvard Medical School,
Boston, Massachusetts, USA*

and

Christopher P. Cannon

*Senior Investigator, TIMI Study Group, Brigham and
Women's Hospital Associate Professor, Harvard
Medical School, Boston, Massachusetts, USA*

WILEY-BLACKWELL

A John Wiley & Sons, Ltd., Publication

This edition first published 2009
© 2009 John Wiley & Sons Ltd.

Wiley-Blackwell is an imprint of John Wiley & Sons, formed by the merger of Wiley's global Scientific, Technical and Medical business with Blackwell Publishing.

Registered office: John Wiley & Sons Ltd, The Atrium, Southern Gate, Chichester, West Sussex, PO19 8SQ, UK

Other Editorial Offices:
9600 Garsington Road, Oxford, OX4 2DQ, UK
111 River Street, Hoboken, NJ 07030-5774, USA

For details of our global editorial offices, for customer services and for information about how to apply for permission to reuse the copyright material in this book please see our website at www.wiley.com/wiley-blackwell

The right of the author to be identified as the author of this work has been asserted in accordance with the Copyright, Designs and Patents Act 1988.

Library of Congress Cataloguing-in-Publication Data

Gelfand, Eli V.
 Management of acute coronary syndromes / Eli V. Gelfand and Christopher P. Cannon.
    p. ; cm.
 Includes bibliographical references and index.
 ISBN 978-0-470-72557-3
 1. Coronary heart disease. 2. Myocardial infarction. I. Cannon, Christopher P.
 II. Title.
 [DNLM: 1. Acute Coronary Syndrome—therapy. 2. Acute Disease—therapy.
 3. Coronary Disease—therapy. WG 300 G316m 2009]
 RC685.C6G45 2009
 616.1'23—dc22

                                                                    2009001962

A catalogue record for this book is available from the British Library.

Set in 10/12 Frutiger by Integra Software Services Pvt. Ltd., Pondicherry, India.
Printed and bound in Great Britain by T.J. International Ltd, Padstow, Cornwall.

First Impression   2009

To Ellen, Sonya and Leah, with love and gratitude.
E.G.

Contents

List of contributors

Christopher P. Cannon, Senior Investigator, TIMI Study Group, Brigham and Women's Hospital, Associate Professor, Harvard Medical School, Boston, Massachusetts, U.S.A.

Jersey Chen, Assistant Professor of Medicine, Department of Internal Medicine, Section of Cardiovascular Medicine, Yale University School of Medicine, New Haven, Connecticut, U.S.A.

Eli V. Gelfand, Director of Ambulatory Cardiology, Beth Israel Deaconess Medical Center, Harvard Medical School, Boston, Massachusetts, U.S.A.

Alena Goldman, Fellow in Cardiac Electrophysiology, Beth Israel Deaconess Medical Center, Harvard Medical School, Boston, Massachusetts, U.S.A.

Jan M. Pattanayak, Fellow in Interventional Cardiology, Beth Israel Deaconess Medical Center, Harvard Medical School, Boston, Massachusetts, U.S.A.

Alisa B. Rosen, Assistant Professor of Medicine, Boston University School of Medicine, Section of Cardiovascular Medicine, Boston Medical Center, Boston, Massachusetts, U.S.A.

Jason Ryan, Assistant Professor of Medicine, Division of Cardiology, University of Connecticut Health Center, Farmington, Connecticut, U.S.A.

Foreword

At an estimated 1.4 million admissions per year, acute coronary syndrome (ACS) is the most common diagnosis of patients with cardiac disease admitted to acute care hospitals in the U.S.A. An even larger number of patients present to emergency departments for evaluation of ACS and to physician offices for out-patient treatment of milder forms of this condition. The prevalence of ACS is growing, not only in the U.S.A. but worldwide, in large measure secondary to the twin epidemics of diabetes and obesity.

ACS covers a broad spectrum of patients, ranging from those with episodes of ischemic chest pain at rest without evidence of myocardial necrosis (unstable angina) to those with cardiogenic shock secondary to ST-segment-elevation myocardial infarction (STEMI). Given its very high prevalence, the diagnostic and therapeutic approaches to ACS must be mastered by cardiologists, primary care physicians, hospitalists, and emergency medicine physicians.

Fortunately, there have been remarkable advances in the diagnosis and assessment of ACS, including new biomarkers and imaging techniques. Likewise, there have been important improvements in therapy, such as new antithrombotic and antiplatelet agents and a more nuanced approach to revascularization therapy. Most of these advances have resulted from large randomized clinical trials.

This excellent handbook summarizes the clinical, diagnostic, and therapeutic aspects of ACS and features valuable sections on special groups of patients, including those with diabetes mellitus and pregnant women. Drs. Gelfand and Cannon and their talented co-authors should be congratulated on the preparation of this handbook. It will be of enormous aid to physicians and trainees who are called upon to care for this ever-increasing number of patients.

Eugene Braunwald
Boston, Massachusetts, U.S.A.

CHAPTER 1
Pathophysiology of acute coronary syndromes

Alisa B. Rosen and Eli V. Gelfand

Introduction

Acute coronary syndromes (ACS) comprise a spectrum of clinical conditions, initiated by rupture of an atherosclerotic coronary plaque with overlying acute thrombosis. The consequences of thrombosis include direct obstruction of blood flow to the coronary beds, as well as distal embolization of the platelet-rich thrombus. Both of these processes may lead to myocardial ischemia and may progress to myocyte necrosis and myocardial infarction. The coronary thrombus may be completely occlusive, as is frequently seen in ST-segment-elevation myocardial infarction (STEMI), or nonocclusive, as can be observed in unstable angina or non-ST-elevation myocardial infarction (UA/NSTEMI). The latter two entities are also known collectively as non-ST-elevation acute coronary syndromes (NSTEACS). This chapter discusses the basic pathophysiology underlying ACS.

Braunwald has described five processes contributing to development of ACS, or any atherothrombotic event (Figure 1.1). These processes include: (1) thrombus on preexisting plaque, (2) dynamic obstruction from coronary spasm or Prinzmetal's angina, (3) progressive mechanical obstruction, (4) inflammation and/or infection, and (5) secondary unstable angina due to global myocardial oxygen supply and demand mismatch.

Management of Acute Coronary Syndromes   Eli V. Gelfand and Christopher P. Cannon
© 2009 John Wiley & Sons, Ltd

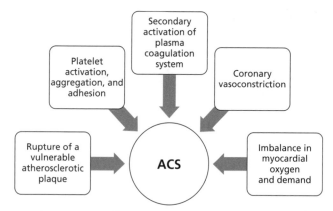

Figure 1.1 Processes contributing to the development of ACS.

Formation of atherosclerotic plaque

Complex plaques of mature atherosclerosis are the end-result of a long pathophysiologic process, which typically begins in early adulthood. Endothelial dysfunction appears to play an initial role in atherosclerosis. Injury to the endothelium results in establishment of the cycle of inflammatory cell migration and proliferation, tissue damage, and repair, and ultimately leads to plaque growth. These mechanisms are outlined in Table 1.1 and are further illustrated in Figure 1.2 (see color plate for a full-color version).

On histological specimens, early precursors of complex plaques include intimal thickening, isolated lipid-containing macrophage foam cells, and pools of extracellular lipids. These are visible on gross specimens as fatty streaks, and

Table 1.1 Primary components of atherosclerotic plaque formation, initiated by endothelial dysfunction (data from Ross[1])

- Increased endothelial adhesiveness
- Increased endothelial permeability
- Migration and proliferation of smooth muscle cells and macrophages
- Release of hydrolytic enzymes, cytokines, and growth factors
- Focal vessel wall necrosis
- Tissue repair with fibrosis

A

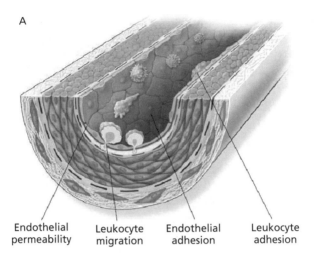

| Endothelial permeability | Leukocyte migration | Endothelial adhesion | Leukocyte adhesion |

B

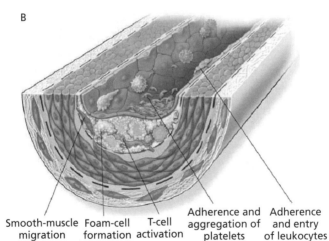

Smooth-muscle migration   Foam-cell formation   T-cell activation   Adherence and aggregation of platelets   Adherence and entry of leukocytes

Figure 1.2 The mechanism of atherosclerotic plaque formation (reproduced from Ross *N Engl J Med* 1999; 340: 115–26). (A) Early endothelial dysfunction in atherosclerosis; (B) fatty streak formation; (C) formation of advanced complex lesion of atherosclerosis; (D) formation of an unstable fibrous plaque. A full-color version of this figure appears in the plate section.

C

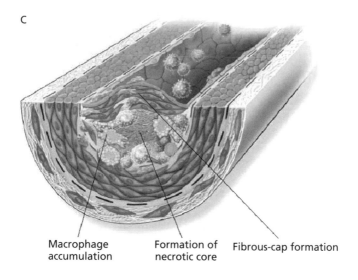

Macrophage   Formation of   Fibrous-cap formation
accumulation   necrotic core

D

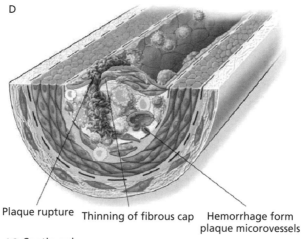

Plaque rupture   Thinning of fibrous cap   Hemorrhage form
                                            plaque micorovessels

Figure 1.2 Continued.

are present in a substantial proportion of young adults who live in the developed world. Eventually, a reactive fibrotic cap and a large lipid core are formed, the lesion may become neovascularized, and calcium is deposited within the plaque (Figure 1.2).

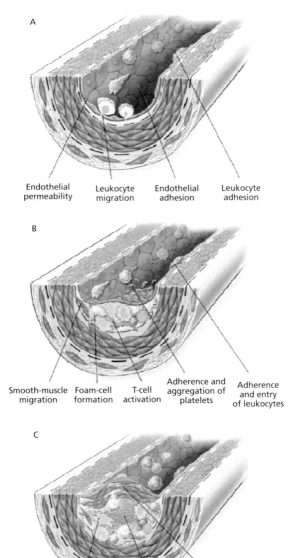

A

Endothelial permeability   Leukocyte migration   Endothelial adhesion   Leukocyte adhesion

B

Smooth-muscle migration   Foam-cell formation   T-cell activation   Adherence and aggregation of platelets   Adherence and entry of leukocytes

C

Macrophage accumulation   Formation of necrotic core   Fibrous-cap formation

Plate 1 The mechanism of atherosclerotic plaque formation (reproduced from Ross *N Engl J Med* 1999; 340: 115–26). (A) Early endothelial dysfunction in atherosclerosis; (B) fatty streak formation; (C) formation of advanced complex lesion of atherosclerosis; (D) formation of an unstable fibrous plaque. See Figure 1.2

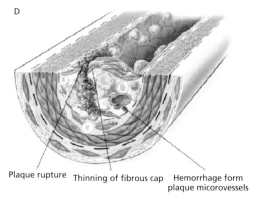

D

Plaque rupture   Thinning of fibrous cap   Hemorrhage form
plaque micorovessels

Plate 1 Continued.

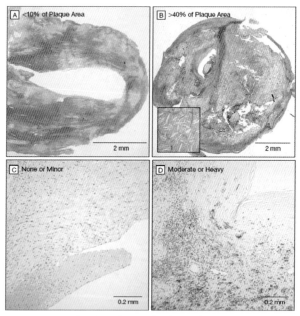

A	<10% of Plaque Area
B	>40% of Plaque Area
C	None or Minor
D	Moderate or Heavy

Plate 2 A representative histology of atherosclerotic plaque (reprinted, with permission, from Hellings *et al. Jama* 2008; 299: 547–54[2]). Collagen staining at low magnification showing fibrous plaque with (A) no lipid core (<10% of the plaque area) and (B) a significant lipid core (>40% of the plaque area) with visible cholesterol crystals (inset). Staining for a macrophage marker CD-68 at higher magnification, demonstrating plaques with (C) minor macrophage infiltration and (D) heavy macrophage infiltration. See Figure 1.3

Plaque instability and the development of ACS

If given enough time, most atherosclerotic plaques gradually progress, although their architecture generally remains stable. Symptoms occur when luminal stenosis reaches 70–80 %. In contrast, the inciting event in the majority of ACS cases is plaque rupture, and most of such plaques occupy <50% of the luminal diameter prior to becoming unstable.[3] Why some plaques rupture and others remain stable for years is incompletely understood, but studies have demonstrated that a large lipid core, a thin fibrous cap, and inflammation within the plaques all predispose to rupture (Figure 1.3 – see color

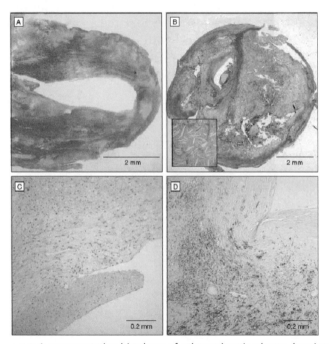

Figure 1.3 A representative histology of atherosclerotic plaque (reprinted, with permission, from Hellings et al. Jama 2008; 299: 547–54[2]). Collagen staining at low magnification showing fibrous plaque with (A) no lipid core (<10% of the plaque area) and (B) a significant lipid core (>40% of the plaque area) with visible cholesterol crystals (inset). Staining for a macrophage marker CD-68 at higher magnification, demonstrating plaques with (C) minor macrophage infiltration and (D) heavy macrophage infiltration (see color plate section for a full-color version).

plate section for full-color version).[4] Inflammation is thought to play a central role in actual plaque disruption.[1] Indeed, a high macrophage content identifies plaques prone to rupture,[5] and unstable, symptomatic plaques can be identified with molecular imaging targeting inflammation.[6] C-reactive protein, a marker of inflammation, is a significant, independent predictor of myocardial infarction, stroke, and peripheral arterial disease.[7]

Exposure of thrombogenic plaque material to flowing blood initiates the endogenous thrombotic response. Actual plaque rupture may precede the clinical syndrome of ACS by several days or even weeks, as evidenced by findings of both fresh and old thrombus in samples of coronary aspirate.[8] It seems likely that most plaque erosions and ruptures are healed with small "sealing" surface thrombi, and major occlusive thrombosis occurs relatively rarely. In these latter cases, however, progressive *in situ*

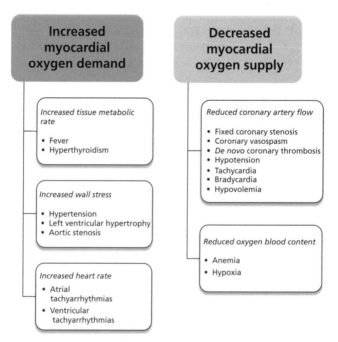

Figure 1.4 Determinants of myocardial oxygen balance and related pathophysiologic factors that contribute to acute coronary syndrome.

thrombosis, together with plaque and thrombus fragment embolization to the distal coronary microcirculation, and the overlying vasospastic response, create conditions for myocardial ischemia.

Myocardial ischemia

Myocardial ischemia occurs when the oxygen demand of the myocardium is greater than its oxygen supply (Figure 1.4). An acute thrombotic coronary occlusion in a previously patent vessel abruptly decreases myocardial oxygen supply. Alternatively, in a patient with a stable intracoronary plaque, elevated heart rate may cause myocardial ischemia by increasing myocardial oxygen demand without having the ability to increase supply. Although most cases of ACS are caused by decreased myocardial oxygen demand, a thorough understanding the components of myocardial oxygen demand and supply is crucial to an understanding of the pathophysiology of myocardial ischemia.

Thrombus formation

Acute coronary syndrome is largely caused by thrombus formation on preexisting plaque. This has been shown through both autopsies and coronary angiography.[9,10] Platelets and the plasma coagulation system are the two major mechanisms through which a thrombus is formed (Figure 1.5).

Platelets

Platelets play a major role in primary hemostasis and in thrombus formation. This occurs in three stages: platelet adhesion, platelet activation, and platelet aggregation (Figure 1.5).[12]

Platelet adhesion
1 Plaque rupture exposes collagen and tissue factor to the bloodstream.
2 GP Ib receptor on platelets interacts with von Willabrand Factor (vWF) to adhere to the damaged endothelial surface.

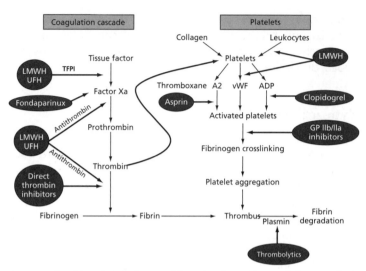

Figure 1.5 An abbreviated schema of thrombus formation and pharmacologic agents targeting thrombosis pathways (adapted, with permission, from Selwyn *Am J Cardiol* 2003; 91: 3H–11H[11]).

Platelet activation
1 Platelet degranulation releases thromboxane A2 (TxA2), adenosine diphosphate (ADP), and other chemoattractants that mediate platelet aggregation. Thrombin and tissue factors also stimulate platelet aggregation.
2 Platelets undergo a conformational change, from a smooth shape to an irregular shape with a larger surface area.
3 Platelets express the GPIIb/IIIa receptor.

Platelet aggregation
1 GPIIb/IIIa receptors on the surface of the activated platelets interact with circulating fibrinogen.
2 Fibrinogen acts as a bridge between GPIIb/IIIa receptors on multiple activated platelets, causing the formation of a platelet plug.
Given that thrombus formation in coronary arteries is the major pathologic process causing ACS, many of the important pharmacologic agents used to treat ACS target platelet function.

Medications that act by interfering with primary hemostasis
1 **Aspirin** inhibits the production of TxA2 by inhibiting cyclooxygenase, an enzyme in the pathway that converts arachadonic acid to TxA2 and other prostaglandins.
2 **Thienopyridines (ticlopidine, clopidogrel, prasugrel)** block the ADP receptor on the platelet, which inhibits platelet aggregation and binding of fibrinogen to the GIIb/IIIa receptor on activated platelets.
3 **GPIb/IIIa receptor antagonists** directly bind to the receptors that mediate platelet aggregation.

Secondary hemostasis

Secondary hemostasis (the **coagulation cascade**) is activated concurrently with the platelet-mediated primary hemostatic mechanisms described above (Figure 1.5). Plaque rupture exposes tissue factor to the bloodstream, which both has a role in platelet adhesion and in activation of the extrinsic system of the clotting cascade.

The production of thrombin
1 Plaque rupture exposes collagen and tissue factor to the bloodstream.
2 Tissue factor converts factor X to Xa.
3 Factor Xa converts prothrombin to thrombin.

The role of thrombin in thrombosis
1 Thrombin converts fibrinogen to fibrin, which is the final step in clot formation.
2 It activates factor XIII, which causes crosslinking of fibrin and stabilization of the clot.
3 It stimulates platelet aggregation (as part of primary hemostasis).

Some medications that act by interfering with the coagulation cascade
1 **Unfractionated heparin** activates antithrombin II (ATII), which inactivates factor Xa and thrombin.
2 **Low molecular weight heparin (LMWH)** also activates antithrombin, which inactivates factor Xa. However, LMWH has a much lesser effect on thrombin than does unfractionated heparin.

3 **Direct thrombin inhibitors (bivalirudin, argatroban)** inhibit thrombin and therefore prevent the conversion of fibrin to fibrinogen.

4 **Factor Xa inhibitor (fondaparinux)** inactivates factor Xa, which then prevents the conversion of prothrombin to thrombin.

In the setting of ACS, the normal balance between thrombosis and endogenous fibrinolysis is disrupted in favor of thrombosis. In addition to medications aimed at inhibiting formation of a platelet plug (aspirin, clopidogrel, GIIb/IIIa receptor antagonists), anticoagulants such as unfractionated heparin, LMWH, direct thrombin inhibitors, and factor Xa inhibitors are beneficial in the treatment of ACS (this is discussed further in Chapters 3 and 4).

Dynamic obstruction

Dynamic obstruction can occur with epicardial coronary vasospasm or be limited to the microcirculation. Symptomatic epicardial vasospasm (Prinzmetal's angina) can occur either at the site of a preexisting nonobstructive atherosclerotic plaque or in a normal portion of the vessel.[13] Nonfocal coronary vasospasm can occur in the setting of cocaine use, cold immersion, or emotional stress.[14,15] Angiographic evidence of epicardial coronary obstruction may be absent if the study is performed at a later time, but recurrent spasm may be demonstrated by asking the patient to hyperventilate on the angiography table. Microcirculatory angina can occur with vasoconstriction in small intramural arteries.

Progressive mechanical obstruction

Progressive mechanical obstruction is an unusual cause of ACS. It is most frequently seen when progressive in-stent restenosis causes decreasing myocardial oxygen supply over the course of months. Gradual-onset exertional angina, not ACS, is a more typical outcome of progressive mechanical obstruction.

Inflammation

As discussed above, inflammation appears to play a major role in initiation and progression of atherosclerosis, as well as in the transition from a stable to an unstable plaque and the onset of acute atherothrombosis.

Secondary unstable angina

Secondary unstable angina is myocardial ischemia/infarction caused by a process other than plaque rupture with thrombus formation. Anemia, bradycardia and severe hypotension are common causes of reduced oxygen supply, whereas tachycardia, fever, and hyperthyroidism frequently increase myocardial oxygen demand. Secondary angina is further discussed in Chapter 5.

References

1. Ross R. Atherosclerosis—an inflammatory disease. *N Engl J Med* 1999; 340: 115–26.
2. Hellings WE, Moll FL, De Vries JP, *et al*. Atherosclerotic plaque composition and occurrence of restenosis after carotid endarterectomy. *Jama* 2008; 299: 547–54.
3. Giroud D, Li JM, Urban P, Meier B, Rutishauer W. Relation of the site of acute myocardial infarction to the most severe coronary arterial stenosis at prior angiography. *Am J Cardiol* 1992; 69: 729–32.
4. Thieme T, Wernecke KD, Meyer R, *et al*. Angioscopic evaluation of atherosclerotic plaques: validation by histomorphologic analysis and association with stable and unstable coronary syndromes. *J Am Coll Cardiol* 1996; 28: 1–6.
5. Fishbein MC, Siegel RJ. How big are coronary atherosclerotic plaques that rupture? *Circulation* 1996; 94: 2662–6.
6. Rudd JH, Warburton EA, Fryer TD, *et al*. Imaging atherosclerotic plaque inflammation with [18F]-fluorodeoxyglucose positron emission tomography. *Circulation* 2002; 105: 2708–11.
7. Ridker PM, Hennekens CH, Buring JE, Rifai N. C-reactive protein and other markers of inflammation in the prediction of cardiovascular disease in women. *N Engl J Med* 2000; 342: 836–43.
8. Rittersma SZ, van der Wal AC, Koch KT, *et al*. Plaque instability frequently occurs days or weeks before occlusive coronary thrombosis: a pathological thrombectomy study in primary percutaneous coronary intervention. *Circulation* 2005; 111: 1160–5.

9. Silva JA, White CJ, Collins TJ, Ramee SR. Morphologic comparison of atherosclerotic lesions in native coronary arteries and saphenous vein graphs with intracoronary angioscopy in patients with unstable angina. *Am Heart J* 1998; 136: 156–63.
10. Nesto RW, Waxman S, Mittleman MA, *et al*. Angioscopy of culprit coronary lesions in unstable angina pectoris and correlation of clinical presentation with plaque morphology. *Am J Cardiol* 1998; 81: 225–8.
11. Selwyn AP. Prothrombotic and antithrombotic pathways in acute coronary syndromes. *Am J Cardiol* 2003; 91: 3H–11H.
12. Kennon S, Price CP, Mills PG, *et al*. The central role of platelet activation in determining the severity of acute coronary syndromes. *Heart* 2003; 89: 1253–4.
13. Kaski JC, Tousoulis D, McFadden E, Crea F, Pereira WI, Maseri A. Variant angina pectoris. Role of coronary spasm in the development of fixed coronary obstructions. *Circulation* 1992; 85: 619–26.
14. Pitts WR, Lange RA, Cigarroa JE, Hillis LD. Cocaine-induced myocardial ischemia and infarction: pathophysiology, recognition, and management. *Prog Cardiovasc Dis* 1997; 40: 65–76.
15. Strike PC, Steptoe A. Systematic review of mental stress-induced myocardial ischaemia. *Eur Heart J* 2003; 24: 690–703.

CHAPTER 2
Diagnosis of acute coronary syndrome

Eli V. Gelfand and Alisa B. Rosen

Introduction

Acute coronary syndromes are associated with significant morbidity and mortality, and thus rapid triage and diagnosis is essential. It is estimated that up to 4% of patients with acute cardiac ischemia are mistakenly discharged from the emergency department, and that these patients have a substantial rate of adverse outcomes.[1] While "typical" symptoms of ACS frequently lead to a prompt diagnosis, a high index of suspicion is required in patients who cannot give an accurate history, including the elderly, and those with significant cardiac risk factors and atypical symptoms, particularly diabetics.

Definition of myocardial infarction

The increasing availability of various laboratory diagnostic tools and sophisticated imaging techniques produces a more detailed and complex matrix of results obtained along the diagnostic ACS pathway. Large numbers of patients present with ACS after having previously undergone coronary revascularization. Adapting to this shifting landscape, several European and U.S. professional societies put forward a set of universal definitions of myocardial infarction (Table 2.1).[2] While acknowledging that ACS also

Table 2.1 Universal definition of myocardial infarction (from Thygesen *et al. Eur Heart J* 2007; 28: 2525–38[2])

Type 1	MI consequent to a pathologic process in the wall of the coronary artery (plaque erosion/rupture, fissuring, or dissection)
Type 2	MI consequent to increased oxygen demand or decreased supply (coronary artery spasm, coronary artery embolus, anemia, arrhythmias, hypertension or hypotension)
Type 3	Sudden unexpected cardiac death before blood samples for biomarkers could be drawn, or before their appearance in the blood
Type 4a	MI associated with PCI
Type 4b	MI associated with stent thrombosis
Type 5	MI associated with coronary artery bypass graft surgery

includes unstable angina (without MI), the guidelines note that the primary difference between UA and MI is that in MI the ischemia is severe enough to cause the release of detectable amounts of cardiac biomarkers.

History

The classic presenting complaint is chest discomfort, which patients often describe as substernal "tightness," "heaviness," or "pressure." It may radiate to the neck, jaw, shoulder, or arm. It may also be associated with shortness of breath, diaphoresis, palpitations, nausea, and lightheadedness (Table 2.2). The examiner should ask what makes the

Table 2.2 Features associated with cardiac chest pain

1 Accompanied by:
   - Shortness of breath
   - Diaphoresis
   - Palpitations
   - Nausea
   - Lightheadedness
2 Radiates to arm, neck, or jaw
3 Is worse with exertion
4 May improve following nitroglycerin administration

discomfort better and worse—cardiac chest pain will generally be exacerbated by exertion and may be relieved by nitroglycerin. On the other hand, historical features, listed in Table 2.3, make it less likely that the discomfort is anginal in nature. It is increasingly recognized that in certain subgroups of patients, including the elderly, women, diabetics, and those with heart failure, the symptoms may be atypical.

Table 2.3 Features of chest pain associated with a low (<3%) likelihood of ACS (from Lee *et al. Arch Intern Med* 1985; 145: 65–9[3])

1 Sharp or stabbing pain
2 No history of angina or MI
3 Pain with pleuritic or positional components, or pain that was reproduced by palpation of the chest wall

The discomfort of ACS must be differentiated from a variety of acute and chronic conditions that may mimic ischemic pain (Table 2.4). In particular, clinicians should be alert to the possibility of acute aortic dissection, since in its presence,

Table 2.4 Differential diagnosis of chest pain

Coronary ischemia (discussed in the text)
Noncardiac life-threatening causes of chest pain:
- **aortic dissection**
  - *Risks*: hypertension, bicuspid aortic valve, Marfan syndrome
  - *Clinical presentation*: chest pain radiating to back, may have hypotension/tachycardia
  - *Physical examination*: unequal brachial blood pressures, diminished pulses in the legs, aortic insufficiency murmur, muffled heart sounds
  - *Diagnosis*: Chest X-ray with widened mediastinum, dissection visualized on CT angiography or TEE
- **pulmonary embolism**
  - *Risks*: cancer, oral contraceptive use, pregnancy, postoperative state, extended period of immobility, hypercoagulable state
  - *Clinical presentation*: pleuritic chest pain, tachycardia, calf pain
  - *ECG*: sinus tachycardia, right heart "strain"
  - *Diagnosis*: elevated D-dimer, pulmonary artery filling defects on CT angiography

Continued

Table 2.4 Continued

- **tension pneumothorax**
  - *Risks*: trauma, COPD, tall stature, recent thoracic surgery
  - *Clinical presentation*: chest pain, hypoxia, hypotension, tachycardia
  - *Physical examination*: absent breath sounds in one lung field
  - *Diagnosis*: CXR will show pneumothorax

Other cardiac causes of chest pain:
- **Pericarditis**
  - *Risks*: may have predisposing viral illness, recent cardiac surgery, connective tissue disease
  - *Clinical presentation*: chest pain, with relief when leaning forward
  - *Physical examination*: may have a pericardial friction rub
  - *ECG*: ST elevation with PR segment depression in most leads, PR segment elevation in aVR
  - *Diagnosis*: clinical
- **Myocarditis**
  - *Presentation and findings*: often similar to acute coronary syndrome, may have heart failure
  - *Cardiac enzymes*: elevated
  - *Echo*: may show global or regional hypokinesis

Common noncardiac cardiac causes of chest pain:
- **GI**
  - esophageal spasm
  - GERD/peptic ulcer disease
  - pancreatitis
  - cholecystitis
- **Musculoskeletal**
  - rib fracture/bruising
  - costrochondritis
  - muscle strain
  - radiculopathy with neck/arm pain
- **Pulmonary**
  - pneumothorax
  - pneumonia/pleurisy
- **Psychiatric**
  - panic attack

treatment with thrombolysis and anticoagulation can lead to catastrophic hemorrhage. Acute pericarditis frequently mimics ACS, and may be associated with chest pain and ST-segment abnormalities on the ECG.

Risk factors

Patients who have known coronary artery disease, and especially those with prior ACS or coronary revascularization, are more likely to have an ischemic cause of their symptoms. Patients with known cerebrovascular or peripheral arterial disease are also more prone to concominant coronary disease.

Patients with prior coronary stent implantation are at risk for stent thrombosis. Stent thrombosis is a sudden thrombotic occlusion of a stent, which most frequently results in transmural ischemia and manifests as severe ischemic symptoms and ST-segment elevations on an ECG. Stent thrombosis is most frequent in the first 30 days following stent implantation, particularly in patients who are noncompliant with antiplatelet therapy. However, late (>30 days after implantation) and very late (>1 year after implantation) stent thrombosis is well-described. Therefore, in patients with prior stent implantation, detailed history of daily compliance with antiplatelet therapy must be elicited. Patients with strong suspicion of stent thrombosis are typically referred for emergent coronary angiography.

In patients without known CAD, it is important to ask whether the classic risk factors for CAD are present (Table 2.5). Cocaine is a powerful precipitant of ACS, and its recent use has specific implications for therapy of ACS (see Chapter 5).

Table 2.5 Cardiac risk factors

- Age (men ≥ 55, women ≥ 65)
- Diabetes
- Smoking
- Hypertension
- Hypercholesterolemia
- Family history of early CAD (men ≤ 55, women ≤ 65)

Physical examination

The physical examination plays an important complementary role in the diagnosis of ACS. It serves to determine the probability of competing diagnoses, as well to assess the severity of ACS (Tables 2.6 and 2.7).

The patient's **general appearance** is often one of the best clues to illness severity in ACS. During episodes of myocardial

Table 2.6 Examination findings suggestive of a diagnosis other than ACS

Absent breath sounds on one side	Pneumothorax
Focal area of consolidation in the lung	Pneumonia
Chest wall tenderness with palpation	Musculoskeletal pain
Reproducible pain with movement of neck or arm	Radiculopathy, shoulder or chest wall pathology
Right upper quadrant tenderness to palpation	Gall bladder etiology
Presence of skin lesions in distribution of pain, along a dermatome	Herpes zoster

Table 2.7 Examination findings suggesting increased risk of adverse outcome

- Hypotension
- Tachycardia or bradycardia
- Presence of third heart sound (S3)
- Pulmonary rales
- New murmur or mitral regurgitation

ischemia, patients may appear pale, clammy, and dyspneic. The classic Levine sign of "fist-to-the-chest" is a finding not sensitive for a diagnosis of ACS, but in the authors' experience, is reasonably specific and observed not infrequently. **Vital signs** in a patients with ACS may disclose both the precipitating cause of the syndrome, such as atrial fibrillation with rapid ventricular rate, or profound hypertension and its consequences. For example, sinus tachycardia may be the earliest manisfestation of impending cardiogenic shock, whereas systemic hypotension despite appropriate initial therapy of ACS may indicate that a large portion of the left ventricle is affected. Sinus bradycardia and heart block may be a sign of inferior infarction in evolution. Hypoxemia measured routinely with noninvasive methods may indicate the onset of pulmonary edema. **Examination of the peripheral vasculature** can point to preexisting noncoronary atherosclerosis. **Neck examination** in particular is often revealing. Indeed, jugular venous pressure (JVP) provides an opportunity to assess right-sided intracardiac filling pressures. Elevated JVP along with peripheral and pulmonary edema argue for total body volume overload, perhaps as a consequence of prior myocardial infarction and congestive heart failure. On the other hand, elevated JVP with clear lungs in the context of ACS can be a sign of right ventricular infarction. **Cardiovascular examination** may disclose an irregular rhythm and prompt a search for atrial fibrillation or ventricular ectopy. The presence of a fourth heart sound as a consequence of acute LV diastolic dysfunction is a frequent finding and is not necessarily a marker of poor outcome. On the other hand, a third heart sound may be a sign of heart failure and is associated with worse outcomes. A systolic murmur may be a preexisting finding from chronic valvular pathology, but in the absence of prior documentation should alert the clinician to the possibility of acute mitral regurgitation (either from ischemic papillary muscle dysfunction or frank papillary muscle rupture) or a ventricular septal defect.

A new loud diastolic murmur of aortic regurgitation is *not* a typical feature of ACS, and should prompt a search for an associated ascending aortic dissection, especially if accompanied by unequal blood pressure measurements between the two brachial arteries. More benign alternative diagnoses can also be suggested on examination of the chest. Indeed, point tenderness to palpation, especially when it reproduces the presenting symptoms, points to a musculoskeletal rather than coronary etiology of the discomfort. A friction rub may be a clue to acute pericarditis. **Pulmonary examination** in ACS also serves to assess the severity of ACS and exclude other diagnoses. Pulmonary edema is a poor prognostic sign in ACS. Absent breath sounds on one side or a focal area of consolidation in the lung, however, point to an alternate diagnosis: pneumothorax and pneumonia, respectively.

Electrocardiography

The pathophysiologic basis of ST segment changes during ischemia

During an episode of ischemia, several electrical properties of the affected myocytes change and result in the alteration of the action potential:

1 Resting membrane potential is lowered.
2 The shape of phase 2 of the action potential is altered.
3 Repolarization occurs earlier and the action potential is shortened.

During transmural ischemia, as seen with STEMI, these changes create a voltage gradient between the endocardial and epicardial surfaces of the heart and cause current to flow, resulting in the upward shift of the systolic ECG component (ST segment) compared to the diastolic component (TP segment). This constitutes the basis of ST-segment elevations in STEMI.

With subendocardial ischemia, as observed during UA/NSTEMI, the current of injury points towards that myocardial layer, and ST segment depressions are seen.

A normal ECG does not exclude ACS, because the ST changes may be subtle, may be masked by baseline abnormalities, or may be transient in time. Thus, when clinical suspicion of ACS persists, it is important to repeat ECGs every 10–15 minutes until a diagnosis is established, or ACS excluded by non-ECG means.

Electrocardiography in ST-elevation MI and identification of the infarct-related artery

During STEMI, the morphology of the QRS complex and the ST segment in the leads, representing the electrical activity of the involved region of the myocardium, goes through characteristic sequential morphologic changes (Figure 2.1):

1 Hyperacute T waves develop.
2 Early ST elevations are observed.
3 ST elevations acquire their typical convex shape.
4 R waves are lost and pathologic Q waves develop in about 75% of patients within hours to days.
5 T-wave inversion is seen.
6 ST segments return to normal configuration.

ST-segment elevations are typical of acute transmural MI, but may also be present in other disorders (Table 2.8). In most cases, differentiation of STEMI from these other pathologies is not difficult on clinical grounds.

Localization of an occluded epicardial artery is an important clinical skill, as it helps to assess the amount of myocardium at risk for necrosis, and can guide decisions pertaining to primary reperfusion therapy. A primer on coronary anatomy can be found in the Appendix, and localization of the general territory affected by the infarction is outlined in Table 2.9.

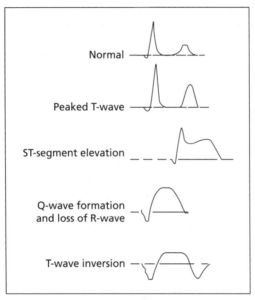

Figure 2.1 The sequence of morphologic changes in ST-segments and T-waves during acute myocardial infarction. Reproduced from Morris F and Brady WJ. Acute myocardial infarction—Part I. *BMJ* 2002; 324: 831–34. Copyright © 2002, BMJ Publishing Group Ltd.

Table 2.8 Causes of ST-segment elevations

Common
- Acute myocardial infarction
- Left ventricular hypertrophy
- Benign early repolarization
- Left bundle branch block
- Acute pericarditis
- Ventricular aneurysm
- Hyperkalemia

Less common
- Acute myocarditis
- Prinzmetal's angina/coronary spasm
- Brugada syndrome
- Subarachnoid hemorrhage
- Hypothermia

Table 2.9 Anatomical relationships of ECG leads

Anterior wall	Leads V_1–V_4
Lateral wall	Leads I, aVL, V_5, and V_6
Inferior wall	Leads II, III, and aVF
Posterior wall	Posterior leads V_7–V_9
Right ventricle	Right-sided chest leads V_1R–V_6R

Anterior MI

An anterior wall MI (AWMI) is caused by the occlusion of the left anterior descending artery (LAD). The ECG of an AWMI will demonstrate ST-segment elevations in leads V_1–V_3 and may show additional ST-segment elevations in leads I and aVL. A simple algorithm allows the location of the occlusion to be determined with respect to the origin of the first diagonal branch (Figure 2.2).[4]

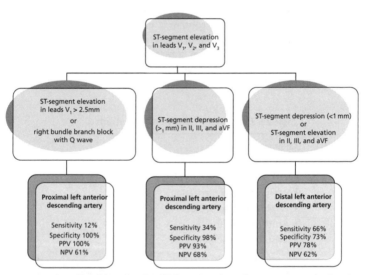

Figure 2.2 An algorithm for localizing the site of coronary occlusion in anterior wall MI (adapted, with permission, from Zimetbaum and Josephson *N Engl J Med* 2003; 348: 933–40[4]).

Left bundle branch block (LBBB) may obscure the ST segment changes of anterior MI, by concealing the activation of the infarcting left ventricle in the terminal portion of a wide QRS complex. However, based on the data from the GUSTO-I trial, inappropriately concordant or extremely discordant changes with the QRS complex were identified as reasonable indicators of an evolving anterior wall MI in the presence of LBBB (Table 2.10).[5]

Table 2.10 Criteria for diagnosis of MI in the presence of LBBB (data from Sgarbossa *et al.*[5])

1 ST-segment elevation $\geq$1 mm in leads with a predominantly positive QRS complex ("inappropriate concordance")

2 ST-segment depression $\geq$1 mm in leads V_1–V_3

3 ST-segment elevation $\geq$5 mm in leads V_1 and V_2 ("extreme discordance")

Inferior MI

Inferior myocardial infarction is caused by occlusion of the right coronary artery (RCA) in 80% of the cases, or the left circumflex artery (LCx) in the rest of the cases. On ECG, ST-segment elevation in leads II, III, and aVF is seen. A simple algorithm allows for differentiation between RCA and LCx as the infarct-related artery (Figure 2.3).

In a patient presenting with an IMI, a search should always be made for a concomitant right ventricular MI, because there are important management and prognostic considerations if the latter is found (see below and Chapter 6).

Posterior MI

Posterior wall MI (PWMI) usually accompanies inferior infarction. The ECG in PWMI demonstrates ST elevation in the inferior leads (II, II, and aVF) and ST segment depression in leads V_1 and V_2.

When there is suspicion for PWMI, additional leads V_7, V_8 and V_9 should be placed on the back (Figure 2.4). If these posterior leads show ST-segment elevation, this offers additional proof of posterior wall involvement.

Right ventricular MI

When there is suspicion for a RVMI, additional leads can be placed on the right side of the chest (Figure 2.5). If there is

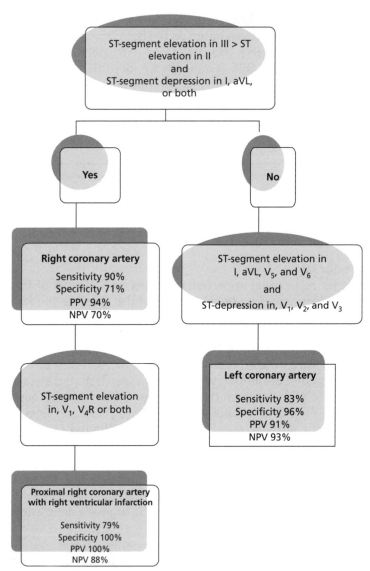

Figure 2.3 An algorithm for localizing the site of coronary occlusion in inferior wall MI (adapted, with permission, from Zimetbaum and Josephson *N Engl J Med* 2003; 348: 933–40[4]).

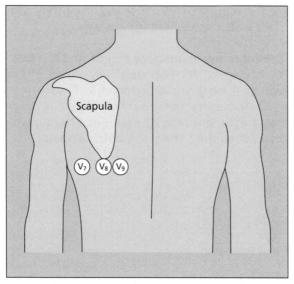

Figure 2.4 The placement of posterior leads for dx of PMI. Reproduced from Morris F and Brady WJ. Acute myocardial infarction—Part I. *BMJ* 2002; 324: 831–34. Copyright © 2002, BMJ Publishing Group Ltd.

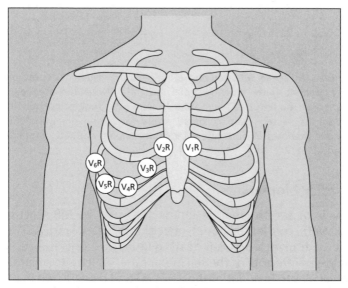

Figure 2.5 The placement of right-sided chest leads. Reproduced from Morris F and Brady WJ. Acute myocardial infarction—Part I. *BMJ* 2002; 324: 831–34. Copyright © 2002, BMJ Publishing Group Ltd.

ST-segment elevation of ≥ 1 mm in V_{4R}, this offers additional proof of RV wall involvement (Chapter 6).

Electrocardiography in unstable angina and NSTEMI

The ECG in UA and NSTEMI classically shows ST segment depression (> 1 mm) and/or symmetric T-wave inversions (Figure 2.6). These changes are more reliable in diagnosing ACS if they are present when the patient is having symptoms and resolve when the patient's symptoms abate.

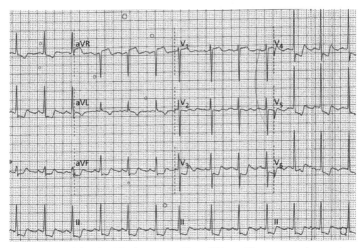

Figure 2.6 A 12-lead ECG, demonstrating diffuse ST segment depressions in a patient with subendocardial ischemia. Note the frequently overlooked finding of ST elevation in lead aVR, suggesting that the patient has a left main coronary artery, or "left-main-equivalent," stenosis (stenoses of both left anterior descending and left circumflex arteries).

Cardiac biomarkers

Levels of serum creatine kinase (CK) and its MB fraction (CK-MB), cardiac troponin, myoglobin, LDH, and AST all rise with myocardial cell death (Figure 2.7). This is a result of loss of integrity of the cell membrane, which allows larger molecules to leak out of the myocyte and be detected in the blood. Myoglobin, CK, LDH, and AST are all elevated in MI, but are not cardiac specific, so their clinical use as a

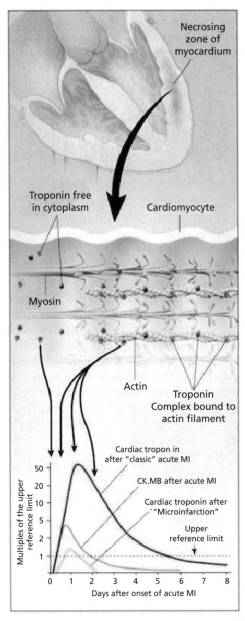

Figure 2.7 The release of cardiac biomarkers in acute myocardial infarction (reproduced, with permission, from Antman *N Engl J Med* 2002; 346: 2079–82[9]).

Table 2.11 Molecular biomarkers for the evaluation of patients with myocardial infarction (data from Antman et al.[6]): cTn = cardiac troponin

Biomarker	Molecular weight	Range of times to initial elevation	Mean time to peak elevation (nonreperfused)	Time to return to normal range
CK-MB	86,000 Da	3–12 h	24 h	48–72 h
cTn I	23,500 Da	3–12 h	24 h	5–10 days
cTn T	33,000 Da	3–12 h	12–48 h	5–14 days
Myoglobin	17,800 Da	1–4 h	6–7 h	24 h

diagnostic tool has waned. The basic characteristics of the common cardiac biomarkers are listed in Table 2.11.

Creatine kinase is a sensitive marker of cardiac muscle death and typically rises within 4–8 hours of MI. However, it is found in skeletal muscle; hence muscle breakdown can also cause elevated CK. For example, CK is typically elevated in rhabdomyolysis, after a crush or electrical injury, or with any type of myositis, and can even be elevated after an intramuscular injection. The MB isoform of CK has high specificity for the myocardium, but is also found in other organs (e.g., the pancreas, placenta, prostate, intestine, diaphragm, tongue, and skeletal muscle). For this reason, the classic definition of MI requires more than a two-fold elevation in total CK with an elevated CK-MB. However, among patients in whom the total CK is normal but a CK-MB fraction is elevated, an increased incidence of death or MI at 6 months has been found.[7]

Troponin is a protein with three subunits (TnI, TnT, and TnC), which controls the interaction between myosin and actin (Figure 2.7). Although TnI and TnT can be found in skeletal muscle, there are antibodies directed specifically against the cardiac forms (cTnI and cTnT), which are highly cardiac specific. Given that the assays are also highly sensitive, cTnI and cTnT are excellent biomarkers for myocardial cell damage, detect even microscopic areas of necrosis, and are increasingly thought to be the preferred cardiac biomarker.[8,9] The 2007 Universal Definition of Myocardial Infarction requires a troponin measurement exceeding the 99th percentile of a normal reference population.[10] Detection of a rise and/or fall of the measurements is essential to the diagnosis of acute myocardial infarction.

Patients presenting with symptoms or an ECG suspicious for ACS may have normal cardiac biomarkers in the first few hours; therefore repeat biomarkers should be obtained in 6–12 hours if clinical suspicion for ACS persists. In STEMI, where reperfusion therapy must be started as soon as possible (Chapter 3), the decision to pursue reperfusion should not be based on initial markers.

Noninvasive imaging

As outlined above, in the majority of cases, the diagnosis of ACS can be arrived at through careful history-taking, physical examination, 12-lead ECG, and laboratory biomarkers. However, in some cases, despite a typical presenting complaint, the physical examination is normal, ECG is unrevealing of ischemic changes, and cardiac biomarkers are normal or borderline. Both established and new imaging modalities then present several excellent choices for making a diagnosis of ACS. They also appear to be particularly useful in identifying those patients with less-than-typical presentation, who are at a *low risk* of having ACS.

Echocardiography

Myocardial ischemia results in focal left ventricular (LV) wall motion abnormality, which is easily identified on a two-dimensional echocardiogram, and *precedes* in its onset both symptoms and ECG abnormalities. In a patient with suspected ACS and a nondiagnostic ECG, obtaining an echocardiogram is recommended by the ACC/AHA/ASE if the study can be obtained during pain or shortly after it ceases.[11] If the echo shows no focal wall motion abnormalities during an episode of chest pain, it is unlikely that ACS is present.[12] An important caveat is that if a focal wall motion abnormality is present in a patient with a history of prior myocardial infarction, distinguishing acute ischemia from an old infarct is difficult.

In addition to confirming or excluding ischemia, resting echocardiography can be useful if it suggests an alternate cause of the patient's symptoms. For example, it may show a pericardial effusion in a case of pericarditis, aortic regurgitation in aortic dissection, or new right ventricular dilation and systolic dysfunction in pulmonary embolism.

Myocardial perfusion imaging

A nuclear perfusion scan while the patient is having chest pain (rest myocardial perfusion imaging) can help assess whether there is a lack of coronary blood flow to a portion of the heart. An ischemic area will show reduced radiotracer counts. This method is difficult to interpret if the patient has had a prior infarct, because reduced radiotracer counts will likewise be observed, even in the absence of acute ischemia.[13]

Coronary computed tomography

Coronary computed tomography (CCT) is rapidly emerging as a powerful imaging tool in patients with suspected ACS. In most cases, complete imaging of the coronary arteries can be performed in under 10 seconds, using less than 10 mSv of radiation exposure and 60–70 ml of iodinated contrast. Off-line reconstruction of the coronary images typically takes another 15–20 minutes. Both calcified and soft plaques are appreciated on CCT (Figure 2.8), although heavy calcification sometimes results in overestimation of the degree of stenosis. In a study of 197 patients presenting to the emergency department with chest pain, the CCT-based diagnostic strategy was compared with the standard of care.[14] CCT was able to exclude or identify coronary disease as a cause of chest pain in 75% of patients, and reduced the time required for diagnosis from 15 hours to under 4 hours. Patients with normal coronary arteries by CCT were discharged immediately, and had fewer repeat evaluations for chest pain than those discharged following conventional evaluation. In patients with mild nonobstructive coronary disease, there is an added incentive to institute aggressive primary prevention measures, including lifestyle modification, glycemic control, antihypertensive and lipid-lowering therapy, and smoking cessation.

Disadvantages of CCT include exposure to ionizing radiation and potentially toxic contrast, as well as its reduced sensitivity in patients with tachycardia and arrhythmia.

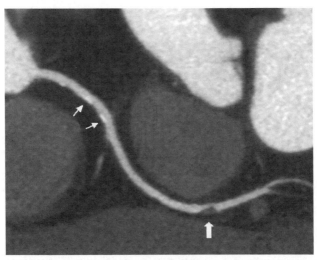

Figure 2.8 A 64-slice coronary computed tomogram in a 46-year-old patient presenting to the emergency department with chest pain. Electrocardiography and cardiac biomarkers were within normal limits. The block arrow shows a hemodynamically *significant soft (noncalcified) plaque* in the mid-segment of the right coronary artery, deemed responsible for this patient's symptoms. Thin arrows point to areas of *nonobstructive calcified plaque* (image courtesy of Milliam Kataoka, M.D.).

Cardiovascular magnetic resonance imaging

Cardiovascular magnetic resonance (CMR) is a gold standard tool for assessing ventricular volumes, mass, and systolic function. It is sensitive in detecting a focal wall motion abnormality. Incorporation of late gadolinium enhancement protocols allows for detection of a perfusion defect and myocardial infarction/scar (Figure 2.9).[15] CMR can also detect an alternative cause for chest discomfort (aortic dissection, pulmonary pathology), depending on the specific protocol and field of view. A CMR examination does not involve the use of ionizing radiation, and that safety of gadolinium-based contrast far exceeds that of iodine-based X-ray contrast agents.

The main disadvantage of CMR is the time required for a study (30–40 min), as well as the inability to image patients with implantable pacemakers or defibrillators.

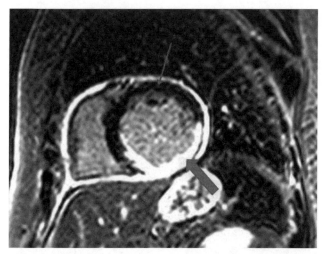

Figure 2.9 A short-axis, mid-ventricular late gadolinium enhancement MRI image in a patient presenting with several days of severe chest pain. There is a large area of dense transmural scar, spanning the inferior, inferoseptal, and inferolateral LV walls (block arrow). Compare with normal-appearing anterior wall myocardium (thin arrow). Based on this image, the likelihood of functional recovery of the infarcted areas is low. Also seen is a small circumferential pericardial effusion.

Stress testing for diagnosis of ACS

Diagnostic stress testing is reserved for patients with possible ischemic symptoms, in whom an initial evaluation, with serial biomarkers and ECGs, does not clearly demonstrate ACS. If no arrhythmia, hemodynamic instability, or recurrent ischemic-type symptoms are present over the course of such an evaluation, stress testing is both safe and valuable. In a study of 1,000 low-risk patients with chest pain, only one instance of myocardial infarction was diagnosed among 582 patients with negative stress testing in the emergency department.[16]

Overall diagnostic pathway for ACS

When a patient presents to the emergency department with symptoms suggestive of acute coronary syndrome (ACS), the general evaluation should proceed through the model of

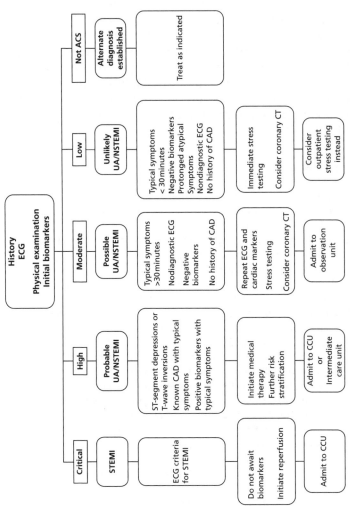

Figure 2.10 A risk-based initial diagnostic pathway: CCU = coronary care.

"stability and initial testing—risk assessment—definite diagnosis or exclusion." Components of this assessment have been outlined in this chapter, and each reader's primary institution is already likely to have a robust pathway in place for efficient diagnosis and management of patients with suspected ACS. One suggested pathway has been initially derived in 1997,[17] and its adapted version is outlined in Figure 2.10. In centers with coronary CT expertise and a reliably short time to image interpretation, both low- and moderate-risk patients may be initially imaged with that modality. Because of concern for cumulative lifetime radiation exposure, however, this strategy is primarily useful in older patients.

References

1. Pope JH, Aufderheide TP, Ruthazer R, et al. Missed diagnoses of acute cardiac ischemia in the emergency department. N Engl J Med 2000; 342: 1163–70.
2. Thygesen K, Alpert JS, White HD. Universal definition of myocardial infarction. Eur Heart J 2007; 28: 2525–38.
3. Lee TH, Cook EF, Weisberg M, Sargent RK, Wilson C, Goldman L. Acute chest pain in the emergency room. Identification and examination of low-risk patients. Arch Intern Med 1985; 145: 65–9.
4. Zimetbaum PJ, Josephson ME. Use of the electrocardiogram in acute myocardial infarction. N Engl J Med 2003; 348: 933–40.
5. Sgarbossa EB, Pinski SL, Barbagelata A, et al. Electrocardiographic diagnosis of evolving acute myocardial infarction in the presence of left bundle-branch block. GUSTO-1 (Global Utilization of Streptokinase and Tissue Plasminogen Activator for Occluded Coronary Arteries) Investigators. N Engl J Med 1996; 334: 481–7.
6. Antman EM, Anbe DT, Armstrong PW, et al. ACC/AHA guidelines for the management of patients with ST-elevation myocardial infarction: a report of the American College of Cardiology/American Heart Association Task Force on Practice Guidelines (Committee to Revise the 1999 Guidelines for the Management of Patients with Acute Myocardial Infarction). Circulation 2004; 110: e82–e292.
7. Galla JM, Mahaffey KW, Sapp SK, et al. Elevated creatine kinase-MB with normal creatine kinase predicts worse outcomes in patients with acute coronary syndromes: results from 4 large clinical trials. Am Heart J 2006; 151: 16–24.
8. Jaffe AS, Ravkilde J, Roberts R, et al. It's time for a change to a troponin standard. Circulation 2000; 102: 1216–20.

9. Antman EM. Decision making with cardiac troponin tests. *N Engl J Med* 2002; 346: 2079–82.

10. Thygesen K, Alpert JS, White HD, *et al*. Universal definition of myocardial infarction. *Circulation* 2007; 116: 2634–53.

11. Anderson JL, Adams CD, Antman EM, *et al*. ACC/AHA 2007 guidelines for the management of patients with unstable angina/ non-ST-Elevation myocardial infarction: a report of the American College of Cardiology/American Heart Association Task Force on Practice Guidelines (Writing Committee to Revise the 2002 Guidelines for the Management of Patients With Unstable Angina/ Non-ST-Elevation Myocardial Infarction) developed in collaboration with the American College of Emergency Physicians, the Society for Cardiovascular Angiography and Interventions, and the Society of Thoracic Surgeons endorsed by the American Association of Cardiovascular and Pulmonary Rehabilitation and the Society for Academic Emergency Medicine. *J Am Coll Cardiol* 2007; 50: e1–e157.

12. Sabia P, Afrookteh A, Touchstone DA, Keller MW, Esquivel L, Kaul S. Value of regional wall motion abnormality in the emergency room diagnosis of acute myocardial infarction. A prospective study using two-dimensional echocardiography. *Circulation* 1991; 84: I85–I92.

13. Klocke FJ, Baird MG, Lorell BH, *et al*. ACC/AHA/ASNC guidelines for the clinical use of cardiac radionuclide imaging—executive summary: a report of the American College of Cardiology/ American Heart Association Task Force on Practice Guidelines (ACC/AHA/ASNC Committee to Revise the 1995 Guidelines for the Clinical Use of Cardiac Radionuclide Imaging). *Circulation* 2003; 108: 1404–18.

14. Goldstein JA, Gallagher MJ, O'Neill WW, Ross MA, O'Neil Bj, Raff GL. A randomized controlled trial of multi-slice coronary computed tomography for evaluation of acute chest pain. *J Am Coll Cardiol* 2007; 49: 863–71.

15. Kwong RY, Schussheim AE, Rekhraj S, *et al*. Detecting acute coronary syndrome in the emergency department with cardiac magnetic resonance imaging. *Circulation* 2003; 107: 531–7.

16. Amsterdam EA, Kirk JD, Diercks DB, Lewis WR, Turnipseed SD. Immediate exercise testing to evaluate low-risk patients presenting to the emergency department with chest pain. *J Am Coll Cardiol* 2002; 40: 251–6.

17. Tatum JL, Jesse RL, Kontos MC, *et al*. Comprehensive strategy for the evaluation and triage of the chest pain patient. *Ann Emerg Med* 1997; 29: 116–25.

CHAPTER 3

Unstable angina and non-ST-elevation myocardial infarction

Eli V. Gelfand and Christopher P. Cannon

Introduction

Of the 1.4 million patients admitted to hospital each year in the U.S. with an acute coronary syndrome, approximately 80% do not have ST-segment elevations on an initial ECG.[1] If serum biomarkers of myocardial necrosis are elevated, these patients are said to have a non-ST-segment elevation myocardial infarction (NSTEMI)—otherwise, unstable angina (UA) is diagnosed. Collectively, these conditions are known as non-ST-segment elevation acute coronary syndromes (NSTEACS).

The American College of Cardiology (ACC) and the American Heart Association (AHA) maintain comprehensive evidence-based guidelines for evaluation and management of UA/NSTEMI,[2] and adherence to these guidelines significantly improves patient outcomes.[3]

Causes of UA/NSTEMI

As described in previous chapters, the typical inciting pathophysiologic event in UA/NSTEMI is erosion or rupture of a vulnerable atherosclerotic plaque, followed by formation of a white, platelet-rich, *nonocclusive* thrombus. The thrombus is inherently unstable, and its fragments embolize downstream, obstructing coronary microvasculature and causing myocardial ischemia. Secondary activation of the plasma coagulation system promotes further thrombosis, and coronary vasoconstriction decreases myocardial oxygen supply, precipitating symptomatic ischemia. When myocardial supply/demand mismatch is severe enough to cause myocyte necrosis, NSTEMI is diagnosed by elevation of cardiac-specific serum biomarkers.

Less common causes of UA/NSTEMI include cardioembolic disease, in which dislodged fragments of a left ventricular intracavitary thrombus or aortic plaque result in partial coronary occlusion, and bacterial endocarditis, where left-sided valvular vegetations may embolize to the coronary circulation. Spontaneous coronary dissection is a relatively uncommon cause of UA/NSTEMI, but should be on the differential diagnosis of ACS in a young woman during pregnancy and peripartum period, and in patients with known connective tissue disease (especially Marfan and Ehlers–Danlos syndromes).

A minority of patients will present with a primary noncardiac condition that effects an oxygen supply/demand mismatch (anemia, thyrotoxicosis, primary arrhythmia, etc.), and will develop symptoms, signs, and electrocardiographic and laboratory evidence of UA/NSTEMI. This is referred to as *secondary unstable angina*[4] or *Type 2 MI*,[5] and is further discussed in Chapter 5.

Presentation of UA/NSTEMI

Patients with UA/NSTEMI typically present with chest discomfort. Unlike in STEMI, where the rest discomfort is classically described as oppressive and unrelenting, in UA/NSTEMI it may be effort-related *or* resting, may vary in severity, and may alternate with angina-free periods. Frequently, such false reassurance of spontaneous anginal relief is a set-up for delayed hospital presentation.

Three general anginal patterns are recognized in UA/NSTEMI. *Rest angina* is a prolonged (>20 min) discomfort during lack of physical activity, and is the typical presentation of NSTEMI. *New-onset angina* refers to newly diagnosed severe discomfort causing marked limitation of physical activity, such as walking one or two city blocks on flat ground, or climbing up a single flight of stairs. *Worsening* angina is diagnosed when previously seen anginal discomfort becomes markedly more intense, prolonged, or brought on by significantly less strenuous activity.[4]

General strategies in management of UA/NSTEMI

Treatment of patients with UA/NSTEMI is directed at preventing recurrent thrombosis via agents directed against formation of thrombin and platelet aggregates, and improving coronary perfusion through selective use of mechanical or surgical revascularization (Table 3.1). Concurrently, myocardial ischemia is managed with antianginal therapy and pain control. Long-term plaque stabilization and secondary prevention of recurrent vascular events is an important early goal, which is achieved through aggressive and evidence-based use of lipid-lowering, antihypertensive, and antidiabetic therapy. Admission with an acute coronary syndrome also presents a unique opportunity to initiate counseling and offer support for smoking

Table 3.1 General strategies for the management of UA/NSTEMI

Prevention of recurrent thrombosis
- *Antiplatelet therapy*: aspirin, clopidogrel, glycoprotein IIb/IIIa inhibitors
- *Antithrombin therapy*: unfractionated or low molecular weight heparins, direct thrombin inhibitors, synthetic pentasaccharide

Improved coronary perfusion
- *Coronary revascularization*: balloon angioplasty, stenting, and adjunctive procedures, coronary artery bypass grafting

Management of ischemia
- *Pharmacologic*: beta-blockers, nitrates, morphine, calcium channel antagonists
- *Mechanical*: intraaortic balloon counterpulsation

Plaque stabilization and secondary prevention
- Treatment of hypertension and dyslipidemia
- Tight glycemic control in diabetic patients
- Smoking cessation, weight reduction, regular exercise
- Therapy for depression and anxiety

cessation, achievement of optimal body weight, and other heart-healthy lifestyle interventions (for more details, see Chapter 7).[2]

Risk stratification of patients with UA/NSTEMI

Patients with UA/NSTEMI encompass a wide range of clinical risk profiles: from those with recent acceleration of anginal symptoms without rest pain or biomarker evidence of myocardial damage, to those with an intermittently occlusive coronary thrombus, marked ST segment changes on a 12-lead ECG, and positive markers of myocardial necrosis (Table 3.2). Risk of death from a UA/NSTEMI ranges from 2.5 to 4.5%, and risk of reinfarction is 2.9–12%, depending on the population studied. Importantly, risk of death and ischemic events remains high even after the index event, and exceeds that of STEMI by about 6 months following presentation.[6] This makes post-discharge care of UA/NSTEMI an integral part of the treatment process. Strategies for

Table 3.2 Measures of increased risk in UA/NSTEMI

Clinical
- Older age
- Diabetes mellitus
- Prolonged or recurrent rest pain
- Congestive heart failure or mitral regurgitation on presentation
- Recurrent ischemia following initial therapy
- Hypotension, bradycardia, tachycardia
- Known extracardiac vascular disease

Electrocardiographic
- Left bundle branch block on presenting ECG
- Persistent $\geq$0.5 mm ST segment depression on presenting ECG
- Transient ST-segment elevations
- Sustained ventricular tachycardia

Laboratory
- Elevated troponin
- Elevated serum creatinine/reduced creatinine clearance
- Elevated BNP or NT-proBNP
- Elevated serum glucose, leucocyte count

secondary prevention of recurrent events after UA/NSTEMI are discussed further in Chapter 7.

Rapid and adaptable risk stratification guides its treatment. Among several formal risk assessment tools for patients with UA/NSTEMI, the **TIMI Risk Score** (TRS; Table 3.3) has been studied most extensively. Developed using the data from the TIMI 11B trial, the TRS is a simple bedside grading system, which utilizes clinical variables already routinely collected by physicians caring for a patient with ACS.[7]

Table 3.3 The TIMI Risk Score for UA/NSTEMI (adapted from Antman et al.[7])

Clinical characteristic (one point each):
- Age ≥65 years
- Prior coronary stenosis >50%
- Three or more conventional CAD risk factors (age, male gender, family history, diabetes, smoking, hypertension, dyslipidemia, obesity)
- Use of aspirin in the preceding 24 hours
- Two or more episodes of angina in the preceding 24 hours
- ST segment deviation (persistent depression or transient elevation)
- Increased cardiac biomarkers

Total TIMI Risk Score: 0–7

In TIMI 11B, the risk of death, MI, or severe ischemia, necessitating urgent revascularization, increased progressively with higher TRS, from <5% for patients with TRS 0–1 to >40% for those with TRS 6–7 (Table 3.4). The TIMI Risk

Table 3.4 The utility of the TIMI Risk Score in predicting short-term adverse events in UA/NSTEMI (data from Antman et al.[7])

TIMI Risk Score	Recurrent MI, severe ischemia, or death at 14 days
0–1	4.7%
2	8.3%
3	13.2%
4	19.9%
5	26.2%
6–7	40.9%

Score has been validated in other clinical trials as well as in the general unselected population of patients with ACS, where it performed equally well.[8] In addition to providing the practicing clinician with rapid means for assessing the patient's short-term risk of adverse events, the TRS defines benefit from specific interventions in UA/NSTEMI, with higher-risk patients deriving benefit from glycoprotein (GP) IIb/IIIA inhibition (vs. placebo), low molecular weight heparin (vs. unfractionated heparin), and invasive (vs. conservative) management strategy.[9–11] The TRS also performs well among patients treated specifically with PCI: higher scores are associated with prolonged hospital stay, higher periprocedural peak troponin levels, and a higher rate of major adverse cardiac events within 30 days of presentation.[12]

Other general measures of increased risk in UA/NSTEMI are listed in Table 3.2. Presenting features such as ischemia-related pulmonary edema, mitral regurgitation, or ventricular tachyarrhythmia define patients at higher risk, and call for expeditious and aggressive therapy.

Initial management of UA/NSTEMI in the emergency department

While the diagnostic work-up is proceeding, and once the diagnosis of UA/NSTEMI becomes established, the ACC/AHA guidelines focus on rapid triage and risk stratification of such patients.[2] This allows for administration of ACS therapies, with proven safety and clinical benefit for a particular patient population.

Initial general measures include the following:
- Twelve-lead ECG within 10 minutes of first contact with a healthcare provider.
- Bed rest.
- Oxygen via nasal cannula.
- Continuous ECG monitoring.
- Close availability of external cardioverter/defibrillator.
- Frequent noninvasive blood pressure monitoring.
- Reliable IV access.
- Chest pain relief with nitrates and morphine (see below).

Pharmacologic treatment of ischemia in UA/NSTEMI

Expeditious relief of ischemia is a important goal in treating UA/NSTEMI. Medications useful for relieving ischemia include beta-blockers, nitrates, morphine, and selected calcium channel blockers (Table 3.5). Systemic hypertension worsens ischemia by contributing to increased ventricular wall stress, and should be treated promptly with

Table 3.5 Anti-ischemic and analgesic therapy in patients with a UA/NSTEMI

Recommended

1 **Nitroglycerin**
   a Sublingual 0.4 mg every 5 minutes until relief of pain (maximum, three doses)
   b Intravenous 10–100 mcg/min for persistent ischemia, heart failure, or hypertension
2 **Beta-blocker** unless contraindicated
   a Metoprolol 25 mg PO, goal heart rate 55–65 bpm, systolic BP 130–140 mmHg
3 **Nondihydropyridine calcium-channel blocker** if beta-blocker contraindicated
   a Verapamil 40–80 mg PO
   b Diltiazem 30–60 mg PO
4 **ACE inhibitor** for patients with LVEF < 40% or pulmonary congestion
   a Captopril 6.25–25 mg PO
   b Enalapril 5–10 mg PO
   c Lisinopril 5–10 mg PO
5 **Morphine sulfate** for persistent ischemic discomfort
6 **Intraaortic balloon counterpulsation (IABP)** for refractory ischemia—because patients typically receive this in the catheterization laboratory, the decision to place IABP is usually combined with the decision to proceed with coronary angiography and revascularization if necessary (see Appendix for IABP primer)

NOT recommended

1 Use of NSAIDs and COX-2 inhibitors for discomfort
2 Use of beta-blockers in patients with signs of acute heart failure or cardiogenic shock, complete heart block, or active asthma flare
3 Use of nitrates in patients with hypotension, bradycardia, or right ventricular infarction
4 Use of nitrates in patients who recently received a phosphodiesterase-5 inhibitor for therapy for erectile dysfunction or pulmonary hypertension (24 hours for sildenafil and vardenafil, 48 hours for tadalafil)
5 Use of immediate-release dihydropyridine calcium channel blockers (e.g., nifedipine)
6 Use of IV ACE inhibitors (e.g., enalaprilat) during the first 24 hours of hospitalization

---

beta-blockers, nitrates, calcium channel blockers, and ACE inhibitors. An adjunctive method for treating severe, refractory ischemia in patients with UA/NSTEMI is placement of an intraaortic balloon pump (IABP). (A primer on IABP may be found in the Appendix.)

Beta-blockers

Beta-adrenergic blockers reduce myocardial contractility, heart rate, and ventricular wall stress, thereby decreasing myocardial oxygen demand and relieving ischemia. Data from randomized clinical trials demonstrate that beta-blockers reduce mortality in ACS.[13] Specifically, among patients with NSTEMI, beta-blocker therapy decreases infarct size and the rate of recurrent MI. Beta-blockers should be administered to all patients with UA/NSTEMI who are able to tolerate it. Contraindications include decompensated congestive heart failure/cardiogenic shock, high-grade atrioventricular (AV) block, severe reactive airway disease, and frank hypotension. Beta-1 selective blockers (**atenolol, metoprolol, bisoprolol**) are preferred to nonselective blockers (**propranolol, nadolol**).

Nitrates

Nitrates reliably result in coronary vasodilation and systemic venodilation, and reduce myocardial oxygen demand. **Nitroglycerin** may be given sublingually at a dose of 0.3–0.6 mg every 5 minutes for up to three doses (Table 3.6). If there is ongoing evidence of ischemia, and particularly if systemic hypertension is also present, intravenous nitroglycerin may be used at doses of 20–200 mcg/min. Close hemodynamic monitoring is required if intravenous nitroglycerin is used. Contraindications to nitrate therapy include systemic hypotension or right

Table 3.6 Nitroglycerin dosage in UA/NSTEMI

	Route	Suggested dosage
Nitroglycerin (NTG)	SL	0.320.6 mg every 5 minutes (maximum, 1.5 mg)
	Buccal spray	0.4 mg every 5 minutes (maximum, 1.5 mg)
	TD	0.2–0.8 mg/h every 8–12 hours
	IV	10–200 mg/min for up to 8 hours

ventricular infarction, as well as co-existing severe aortic stenosis. Patients who use phosphodiesterase-5 (PDE-5) inhibitors within the preceding 24 hours (or 48 hours in the case of tadalafil) should not be given nitrates, as they may precipitate severe, life-threatening hypotension. Nitrates should also not be used in patients with severe tachycardia, bradycardia or hypotension.

Calcium channel blockers

Calcium channel blockers (CCB) are direct coronary vasodilators. **Diltiazem** and **verapamil** are negative inotropes, whereas dihydropyridine-type CCBs (nifedipine, amlodipine, felodipine) are not. Coronary vasodilation as well as a decrease in heart rate produced by diltiazem or verapamil results in reduction of myocardial ischemia by CCB. An early study demonstrated lower incidence of reinfarction among patients with NSTEMI when diltiazem was used.[14] Analysis of several randomized controlled trials of CCB in ACS (with or without ST elevations) shows that on the whole these agents do not reduce the risk of initial or recurrent infarction, or death in ACS,[15] although more recent studies with amlodipine in patients with CAD and hypertension have suggested some clinical benefit. At the present time, the use of long-acting *nondihydropyridine type CCBs* (diltiazem and verapamil) in UA/NSTEMI is reserved for two situations:

1 In the setting of continuing or recurrent ischemia in patients for whom beta-blocker therapy is contraindicated.
2 For ongoing ischemia, when beta-blockers and nitrates are fully employed (long-acting verapamil or diltiazem, amlodipine, felodipine).

Use of short-acting dihydropyridine CCB (**nifedipine**) should be *avoided* in UA/NSTEMI, as the resultant reflex tachycardia increases myocardial oxygen demand, and worsens ischemia. This is especially notable if beta-blockers are not being utilized.

Angiotensin-converting enzyme inhibitors

Therapy with angiotensin-converting enzyme (ACE) inhibitors within the first 24 hours is a Class I indication in patients with UA/NSTEMI who have LV dysfunction and/or congestive heart failure, in absence of hypotension.[2] Extrapolation of the results of HOPE and EUROPA trials of patients with *stable* coronary artery disease, showing a significant reduction in death, MI, and stroke in that population, led to a Class IIa recommendation for ACE inhibitors in all other patients with UA/NSTEMI in the absence of hypotension or a specific contraindication.[16,17] A low-dose, short-acting agent (e.g., captopril 6.25 mg three times per day) is typically administered first, and the patient is observed for hypotension. The dose is then escalated as tolerated, and the patient is switched to an equivalent dose of a longer-acting preparation (lisinopril, quinapril, ramipril, etc.).

Morphine
Small doses of **morphine sulfate** may be administered to patients with continued ischemic chest discomfort despite therapy with nitroglycerin. In addition to reliable analgesia, effects of morphine include significant venodilation, mild arteriolar dilation, and a slight decrease in heart rate, leading to a decrease in myocardial oxygen demand. The drug is particularly useful in patients with pulmonary edema complicating UA/NSTEMI. The suggested dosage of morphine sulfate is 2–5 mg IV every 5–30 minutes, titrated to pain relief. Patients should be monitored carefully for development of respiratory depression. Hypotension may develop on the background of aggressive morphine therapy, particularly if the patient is hypovolemic.

Oxygen
Oxygen should be given to patients who are hypoxemic; however, there are no data supporting prolonged oxygen therapy in *all* patients with UA/NSTEMI.

Invasive versus conservative strategy

The term **early invasive strategy** generally refers to coronary angiography and percutaneous coronary intervention shortly (usually, within the first 4–48 hours) after presentation with symptoms of UA/NSTEMI (Figure 3.1). **Conservative strategy** encompasses antiplatelet, anticoagulant, and anti-ischemic management with medications, often

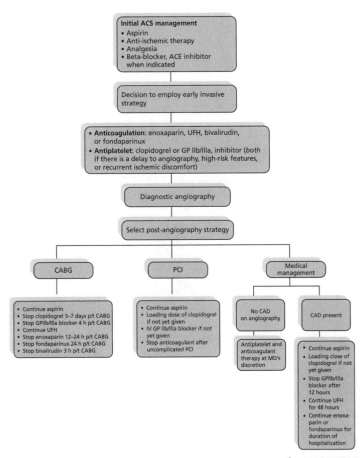

Figure 3.1 An overall **early invasive management** strategy for UA/NSTEMI (adapted from Anderson *et al.*[2]).

followed by functional evaluation, such as stress testing and/ or echocardiography (Figure 3.2). Conservative management strategy does not exclude angiography; the latter is performed for recurrent ischemia, frequent ventricular arrhythmia, hemodynamic instability, or high-risk findings on noninvasive testing. Proponents of early invasive strategy point to the advantages of early identification of high-risk patients who benefit from PCI or CABG. The potential

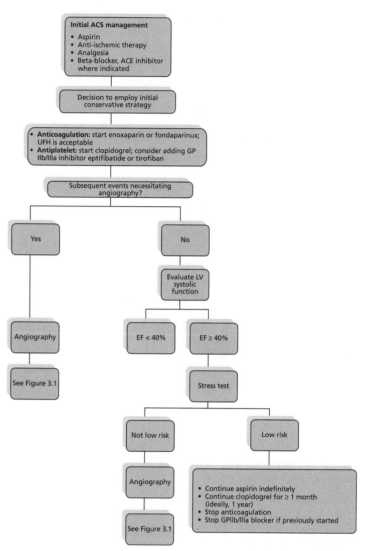

Figure 3.2 An overall **conservative management** strategy for UA/NSTEMI (adapted from Anderson *et al.*[2]).

advantages of the initial conservative strategy include identi-fication of *low-risk* patients, who would not incur a survival or quality-of-life benefit from revascularization, as well as potential cost savings.

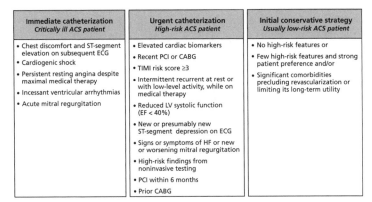

Immediate catheterization *Critically ill ACS patient*	Urgent catheterization *High-risk ACS patient*	Initial conservative strategy *Usually low-risk ACS patient*
• Chest discomfort and ST-segment elevation on subsequent ECG • Cardiogenic shock • Persistent resting angina despite maximal medical therapy • Incessant ventricular arrhythmias • Acute mitral regurgitation	• Elevated cardiac biomarkers • Recent PCI or CABG • TIMI risk score ≥3 • Intermittent recurrent at rest or with low-level activity, while on medical therapy • Reduced LV systolic function (EF < 40%) • New or presumably new ST-segment depression on ECG • Signs or symptoms of HF or new or worsening mitral regurgitation • High-risk findings from noninvasive testing • PCI within 6 months • Prior CABG	• No high-risk features or • Few high-risk features and strong patient preference and/or • Significant comorbidities precluding revascularization or limiting its long-term utility

Figure 3.3 Timing of referral to the catheterization laboratory in patients with UA/NSTEMI.

The decision on whether to refer a patient with UA/NSTEMI to the catheterization laboratory is largely clinically driven (Figure 3.3), although extensive trial-derived data are available to guide the clinician. A number of large randomized trials compared invasive and conservative strategies in patients with UA/NSTEMI (Table 3.7). The majority clearly demonstrated an advantage to early invasive therapy in patient populations at moderate-to-high risk for nonfatal MI, heart failure, or death. The population studied was broad in their presentation: NSTEMI in VANQWISH and VINO trials, UA *or* NSTEMI in the rest of the studies. Markers of increased risk differed slightly between the trials, and included age in TIMI IIIb, elevated serum troponin in FRISC II and TACTICS-TIMI 18, and ST depression in TIMI IIIB, FRISC II, and TACTICS-TIMI 18.

In its 2007 guidelines, the ACC/AHA gave Class I recommendation to early invasive strategy for UA/NSTEMI patients with high risk indicators (Table 3.8).

Antiplatelet therapy in UA/NSTEMI

Antiplatelet therapy is the cornerstone of ACS management; Table 3.9 illustrates the 2007 ACC/AHA guidelines, and individual therapies are discussed below in greater detail.

Table 3.7 Early invasive versus conservative strategy for the management of UA/NSTEMI

Trial	n	Baseline treatment	Time to revascularization in invasive arm	Results	Comments
TIMI IIIB[18]	1,473	tPA vs. placebo (also randomized), ASA, BB, UFH	18–48 hours	No difference in death and MI at 6 weeks (7.5% vs. 8.2%) or 1 year (10.8% vs. 12.2%)	
VANQWISH[19]	920	ASA, BB, UFH, ± fibrinolysis (for STEMI)	>72 hours	*Higher* rate of death or MI at with invasive approach (7.8% vs. 3.2%). Similar outcomes at 2 years after presentation	Patient population limited to non-Q-wave MI only. Patients with a TIMI Risk Score of 5–7 actually benefited from early invasive strategy
MATE[20]	210	ASA, BB, UFH	Mean, 27 hours	Lower incidence of death or recurrent ischemia in the hospital with invasive strategy (13% vs. 34%). No benefit by 21 months	37% rate of revascularization in the *conservative* group (vs. 58% in invasive group)
FRISC II[21]	2,457	ASA, BB, dalteparin	7 days	Lower rate of death/MI in the invasive group (9.4% vs. 12.1%). Difference in mortality not significant at 6 months (1.9% vs. 2.9%) but significant at 1 year (2.2% vs. 3.9%)	Per 1,000 patients, invasive strategy saved 17 lives, and prevented 20 MIs and 20 readmissions for ACS

	N	Therapy	Timing	Results	Comments
VINO[22]	131	ASA, BB, heparin	≤24 h; mean, 6.2 hours	Lower rate of death or MI at 6 months with early invasive strategy (6% vs. 22%)	40% rate of revascularization in the conservative strategy group. Patient population limited to NSTEMI only
TACTICS-TIMI 18[23]	2,220	ASA, BB, UFH, tirofiban	4–48 hours	Lower incidence of combined endpoint of death, MI, or readmission for ACS by 6 months with an invasive strategy (15.9% vs. 19.4%). No mortality benefit from invasive strategy 30 days or 6 months	• Reduction in endpoint with invasive strategy seen overall, with greater benefit in patients with elevated troponin, ST deviation, or TIMI Risk Score ≥ 3 • In women, benefit of invasive strategy also seen among those with elevated troponin
RITA 3[24]	1,810	ASA, BB, enoxaparin	≤72 hours	Lower incidence of death/MI/refractory angina with invasive strategy (9.6% vs. 14.5%). Significant decrease in MI defined by increased troponins at 1 year (9.4% vs. 14.1%)	

Continued

Table 3.7 Continued

Trial	n	Baseline treatment	Time to revascularization in invasive arm	Results	Comments
ISAR COOL[25]	410	ASA, clopidogrel, UFH, tirofiban	Immediate, ≤ 6 hours (median, 2.4 hours) vs. invasive, 4–5 days	Lower incidence of death or large MI at 30 days with *very early* invasive strategy (5.9% vs. 11.6%)	Benefit was due to reduced incidence of events prior to catheterization, whereas there was no difference in events after diagnostic catheterization
ICTUS[26]	1,200	ASA, enoxaparin, abciximab	<48 hours	No difference in mortality (2.5%, both groups), MI more frequent in invasive group (15% vs. 10%), rehospitalization more frequent in conservative group (10.9% vs. 7.4%)	Definition of MI includes CK elevation to 1–2 times upper limit of normal, which does not match the universal definition of MI, and thus handicaps the invasive arm

Table 3.8 ACC/AHA recommendations for early conservative versus invasive strategies in patients with UA/NSTEMI (adapted from Anderson et al.[2])

Class I (definitely recommended)

1 An early invasive strategy is indicated in UA/NSTEMI patients who have refractory angina or hemodynamic or electrical instability

2 An early invasive strategy is indicated in initially stabilized UA/NSTEMI patients who have an elevated risk for clinical events

Class IIb (benefit from therapy less established)

1 In initially stabilized patients, an initially conservative strategy may be considered as a treatment strategy for UA/NSTEMI patients who have an elevated risk for clinical events; this decision can be made by considering physician and patient preference

2 An invasive strategy may be reasonable in patients with chronic renal insufficiency

Class III (not recommended)

1 An early invasive strategy is not recommended in patients with extensive comorbidities (e.g., liver or pulmonary failure, cancer), in whom the risks of revascularization and comorbid conditions are likely to outweigh the benefits of revascularization

2 An early invasive strategy is not recommended in patients with acute chest pain and a low likelihood of ACS

3 An early invasive strategy should not be performed in patients who will not consent to revascularization

---

Table 3.9 ACC/AHA recommendations for antiplatelet therapy in UA/NSTEMI (adapted from Anderson et al.[2])

Class I (definitely recommended)

1 Aspirin (ASA) is the preferred first antiplatelet

2 Clopidogrel (loading dose followed by maintenance dose) is given to hospitalized patients who are unable to take ASA

   a When an *initial conservative strategy* is planned, clopidogrel is given *in addition* to aspirin and anticoagulant

   b When an *early invasive strategy* is planned, clopidogrel *or* a GP IIb/IIIa inhibitor should be given in addition to aspirin before angiography

3 Clopidogrel is continued for at least 1 month and ideally for up to 1 year (and at least a year after DES), and should be withheld for 5–7 days prior to CABG; aspirin should be continued during this time

4 In patients with a history of gastrointestinal bleeding, drugs to minimize the risk of recurrent bleeding should be given to patients taking ASA or clopidogrel

---

Continued

Table 3.9 Continued

5 For all patients, anticoagulation, in addition to antiplatelet therapy, with sub-cutaneous low molecular weight heparin (LMWH), intravenous unfractionated heparin (UFH), or fondaparinux (or bivalirudin as another choice for an invasive strategy) should be given as soon as possible after admission

Class IIa (weight of evidence or opinion is in favor of benefit from therapy)

1 When an *invasive strategy* is planned, GP IIb/IIIa inhibitor and clopidogrel may be given together, in addition to ASA

2 As part of the *initial conservative strategy,* a GP IIb/IIIa inhibitor may be *added to* aspirin, heparin, and clopidogrel in patients who have recurrent ischemic discomfort and are then scheduled for diagnostic angiography

3 When bivalirudin is used as the anticoagulant before angiography, upstream GP IIb/IIIa inhibitor may be omitted as long as aspirin or clopidogrel (300 mg) were administered at least 6 hours before the procedure

Class IIb (benefit from therapy less established)

1 Eptifibatide or tirofiban, in addition to ASA, clopidogrel, and anticoagulant, in patients without continuing ischemia in whom PCI is not planned

Class III (not recommended)

1 Abciximab administration in patients in whom PCI is not planned

Aspirin

Aspirin therapy has an AHA/ACC Class I indication in UA/NSTEMI (Table 3.9).[2] An initial dose of 160–325 mg PO is appropriate, followed by indefinite therapy with 75–162 mg PO daily. Data for aspirin therapy in UA/NSTEMI come from several randomized clinical trials, which were pooled in the Antithrombotic Trialists' Collaboration.[27] This review included over 5,000 patients with UA/NSTEMI enrolled in 12 trials, and treated with antiplatelet therapy, mostly with aspirin. The combined endpoint of MI, stroke, or death from cardiovascular cause was reduced by 46% in patients treated with antiplatelet therapy, compared with placebo.

As reflected by the TIMI Risk Score, development of ACS despite chronic aspirin portends worse outcomes.[7] This apparent paradox is likely a reflection of more widespread atherothrombosis, which "breaks through" *despite* aspirin therapy. A small subset of these patients may have aspirin resistance, testing for which is available in the clinical setting.

Although safe in general, aspirin is associated with an increase in bleeding. Intracranial or life-threatening GI bleeding is rare with aspirin monotherapy even at high doses (<1%), but minor mucosal and GI bleeding is occasionally seen. Data from the CURE and BRAVO trials demonstrated lower bleeding rates with lower aspirin doses; that is, 75–100 mg daily versus 200–325 mg daily.[28,29]

Contraindications to aspirin therapy include active life-threatening bleeding, and true aspirin allergy; that is, urticaria and/or bronchoconstriction. Clopidogrel (see below) may be used in lieu of aspirin for patients with true allergy. Subsequent aspirin desensitization under controlled conditions may permit use of aspirin long-term for secondary prevention.[30] A commonly used protocol is outlined in the Appendix.

Clopidogrel

Clopidogrel at a loading dose of 300 mg by mouth, and a maintenance dose of 75 mg daily, should be administered to most eligible patients with non-ST-elevation ACS (see Table 3.9).[2] Clopidogrel blocks ADP receptors on platelets, thus inhibiting platelet activation and in turn aggregation, and reducing blood viscosity. It was initially studied in the CAPRIE trial, for secondary prevention in a broad range of patients with atherosclerotic heart disease. Compared to aspirin, clopidogrel resulted in an 8.7% relative reduction in long-term combined endpoint of stroke, MI, or cardiovascular death.[31] Dual antiplatelet therapy with clopidogrel and aspirin in non-ST-elevation ACS was addressed in the CURE trial, and the related PCI-CURE study (Table 3.10).

In the CURE trial, patients with UA/NSTEMI were randomized to receive aspirin alone, or aspirin plus clopidogrel, in addition to other standard treatment. The primary endpoint of cardiovascular death, MI, or stroke through follow-up (mean, 9 months; maximum, 1 year) was reduced by 20%, from 11.4% to 9.3%. The benefit of dual antiplatelet therapy continued out to 1 year.[29]

The PCI-CURE study studied the subset of CURE patients who underwent percutaneous revascularization. Pretreatment with clopidogrel reduced the primary endpoint from 6.4% for placebo to 4.5% for clopidogrel—a

Table 3.10 The CURE and PCI-CURE trials

Name	Population	Results
CURE[29]	12,562 patients with UA/NSTEMI randomized to aspirin vs. clopidogrel	20% relative reduction (11.4% to 9.3%) in primary endpoint of cardiovascular death, MI, or stroke through 9 months: • Benefits seen in all subgroups: high or low TIMI Risk Score, present or absent ECG changes, positive or negative cardiac biomarkers • Benefit seen as early as 2 hours after randomization
PCI-CURE[32]	A subset of 2,658 patients from CURE, treated with percutaneous intervention	30% reduction in CV death, MI, or stroke by 30 days after PCI (6.4% to 4.5%) in group treated with clopidogrel prior to PCI

30% relative reduction. The endpoint of cardiovascular death or MI was reduced from 4.4% to 2.9%, a 34% risk reduction.[32]

Clopidogrel is associated with fewer serious side effects than an earlier platelet ADP receptor blocker **ticlopidine**. Neutropenia and thrombotic thrombocytopenic purpura (TTP), which are seen with ticlopidine therapy, are both extremely rare during clopidogrel therapy (four cases per million for TTP). Therefore, routine hematologic follow-up is not mandatory when using clopidogrel.

Data from the CAPRIE trial suggest that clopidogrel mono-therapy is associated with less gastrointestinal bleeding, compared to aspirin.[31] However, dual antiplatelet therapy predictably leads to more hemorrhage. In CURE, the combination of clopidogrel plus aspirin was associated with a relative 35% increase in major bleeding, but the absolute increase was only 1% and there was not an increase in intracranial hemorrhage rate.[29]

Inhibition of platelet aggregation is seen as early as 2 hours after the first dose, and in the CURE trial, benefits of clopidogrel were seen 3 hours after administration.[29] In PCI-CURE, benefits of *pretreatment* with clopidogrel prior to percutaneous intervention were associated with a 30% decrease in the primary endpoint of cardiovascular death, MI, or stroke (Table 3.10).[32]

Patients undergoing CABG within 5 days of treatment with clopidogrel have increased perioperative bleeding. In this subset of patients from CURE, 9.6% of patients treated with clopidogrel had significant bleeding, defined as receipt of ≥ 2 units of blood, compared to 6.3% of patients treated with aspirin alone. However, there was no difference in TIMI major bleeding, and significant benefit was seen in patients treated with CABG including decreases in death, nonfatal MI, and stroke. If surgery was postponed beyond 5 days of clopidogrel treatment, no excess bleeding over aspirin monotherapy was seen. Whether or not to safely operate on a patient who has received clopidogrel within the prior 5 days is often based on the experience of a particular cardiac surgeon, so it is helpful to become familiar with the preference of the surgical department at one's institution when referring patients for coronary bypass grafting.

If patients are treated using a conservative strategy, clopidogrel is continued along with aspirin for 1 year ideally. Pretreatment with clopidogrel also improves outcomes if an invasive strategy with coronary angiography and percutaneous intervention is employed. Following coronary stenting, clopidogrel markedly reduces the risk of stent thrombosis; therefore, prior to the discharge from the hospital, the physician *must* explain to the patient the importance of uninterrupted clopidogrel therapy.[33,34] The length of mandatory therapy with clopidogrel after stenting is determined by the type of stent employed (for more information, see Chapter 7).

Prasugrel

Prasugrel is a novel thienopyridine, with more rapid onset and more potent platelet inhibition than clopidogrel. Approved for clinical use in Europe, the drug is currently undergoing Phase 3 clinical studies in the U.S. and is likely to be approved there shortly. The TRITON-TIMI 38 trial, which included 13,562 patients with ACS (>10,000 with UA/NSTEMI) undergoing planned PCI, compared prasugrel with clopidogrel on the background of aspirin therapy.[35] The primary endpoint of death from cardiovascular causes, nonfatal MI, or nonfatal stroke was reduced by 19% in the prasugrel group, compared with clopidogrel (9.9% vs. 12.1%, respectively). This was partially offset by a higher rate of major bleeding with prasugrel (2.4% vs. 1.8% for clopidogrel). The rate of stent thrombosis was reduced by 52% in the prasugrel group (1.1% vs. 2.4% for clopidogrel).

Glycoprotein IIb/IIIa inhibitors

GP IIb/IIIa inhibitors are useful in patients with UA/NSTEMI, particularly if early invasive strategy is employed. These agents reduce the rate of death, MI, or recurrent ischemia, and lead to a more complete resolution of intracoronary thrombus, as well as improved coronary flow compared with aspirin and heparin alone.[36] The benefit is primarily seen in high-risk patients: those with positive troponin, a TIMI Risk Score of ≥ 4, or ongoing ischemic discomfort. Current ACC/AHA guidelines, therefore, recommend using an intravenous GPIIb/IIIa inhibitor, along with aspirin, clopidogrel, and unfractionated heparin or LMWH, in patients with UA/NSTEMI in whom catheterization with PCI is planned. In patients who are triaged directly to coronary angiography, the drug is often started during the procedure, but if there is a delay between the time of diagnosis and planned PCI, a GPIIb/IIIa inhibitor should be started promptly. Use of **eptifibatide** or **tirofiban** for high-risk patients treated conservatively is also endorsed (Table 3.9), whereas the use of **abciximab** for that indication is discouraged.[2]

Data for intravenous GPIIb/IIIa inhibitors in UA/NSTEMI come from several moderate-sized randomized trials, which are summarized in Table 3.11. A meta-analysis of six trials which included >31,000 patients with UA/NSTEMI who were not scheduled to undergo early routine revascularization demonstrated a significant reduction in death and MI at 5 days (5.7% vs. 6.9%) and 30 days (10.8% vs. 11.8%).[37] Importantly, the benefit was largely limited to patients who underwent PCI or CABG within 30 days, and only to those patients, in whom the troponin I or T concentration was >0.1 ng/ml. GPIIa/IIIb blockers are powerful inhibitors of platelet aggregation, and administration of these agents is associated with a higher rate of major

Table 3.11 Major trials of IV GPIIb/IIIa antagonists in UA/NSTEMI

Rx	Trial	Setting	n	Major results
Abciximab	EPIC[38]	Unstable angina or acute MI treated with PCI	2,099	Significant 35% reduction in death, recurrent MI, CABG, or emergency repeat revascularization at 30 days with abciximab
	EPILOG[39]	Elective or urgent PCI	2,792	Significant 55% relative reduction in death, MI, or urgent revascularization with abciximab
	EPISTENT[40]	Elective or urgent PCI	2,399	Significant 51% relative reduction in death or MI between stenting + placebo and stenting + abciximab groups
	CAPTURE[41]	Refractory unstable angina treated with PCI	1,265	Significant 29% relative reduction in death, MI, and revascularization at 30 days with abciximab
	GUSTO IV-ACS[42]	Unstable angina or NSTEMI—*PCI not planned*	7,800	No significant difference in death or MI at 30 days between abciximab and placebo groups
Eptifibatide	ESPRIT[43]	Elective, urgent PCI (double-bolus of eptifibatide vs. placebo)	2,064	Significant 37% relative risk reduction in primary endpoint of death, MI, and target vessel revascularization at 12 months (6.4% vs. 10.5%)

Continued

Table 3.11 Continued

Rx	Trial	Setting	n	Major results
	IMPACT II[44]	Elective, urgent, emergency PCI	4,010	Nonsignificant benefit of eptifibatide over placebo in reducing death, MI, or urgent revascularization at 30 days
	PURSUIT[45]	Unstable angina or NSTEMI (PCI not mandated)	10,948	Significant reduction in death or nonfatal MI at 30 days with eptifibatide (1.5% absolute reduction)
Tirofiban	RESTORE[46]	Unstable angina or MI with PCI within 72 hours of presentation	2,141	Nonsignificant 16% relative reduction in death, MI, or repeat revascularization at 30 days
	PRISM[47]	Unstable angina or MI with chest pain within *24 hours* (PCI *discouraged* during 48 hours of drug infusion)	3,232	Significant 32% relative reduction in death, MI, or refractory ischemia at 48 hours with tirofiban
	PRISM-PLUS[48]	Unstable angina or MI with chest pain within *12 hours* (PCI *discouraged* during 48 hours of drug infusion, *encouraged* at 48–96 hours)	1,915	Significant 28% relative reduction in death, MI, or refractory ischemia at 7 days with tirofiban; also, significantly lower rate of composite endpoint at 30 days

bleeding: 2.4% versus 1.4% in a meta-analysis.[37] Care must be exercised when small-molecule GPIIb/IIIa inhibitors (eptifibatide or tirofiban) are used in patients with renal insufficiency, as these compounds are renally cleared. In patients with creatinine clearance <50 ml/min, the maintenance infusion of tirofiban must be reduced by one-half. The use of half-dose infusion of eptifibatide is recommended for patients with creatinine between 2.0 and 4.0 mg/dl, and its use is discouraged in patients with creatinine over 4.0 mg/dl. On the other hand, the monoclonal antibody abciximab may be used in patients with renal insufficiency, including those on hemodialysis. Another important adverse effect of GPIIb/IIIa inhibitor therapy is thrombocytopenia, the incidence of which ranges from 0.2% to 2% in clinical trials. Routine measurement of platelet count is indicated prior to initiation of GPIIb/IIIa therapy, 6–8 hours later, and daily thereafter until the infusion is terminated. Treatment of thrombocytopenia in this situation includes cessation of IIb/IIIa therapy, and close observation for bleeding complications. Platelet transfusions are reserved for profound thrombocytopenia (platelet count $<10{,}000/mm^3$) or clinically significant bleeding.

Several *oral* GPII/IIIa inhibitors were evaluated in RCTs, and were found to increase bleeding risk and/or mortality in patients with ACS. Those drugs are, therefore, *not* currently approved for clinical use.

Anticoagulant therapy in UA/NSTEMI

An important aspect of the pathophysiology of UA/NSTEMI involves the release of tissue factor from the ruptured plaque and subsequent activation of the plasma coagulation system, with generation of factor IIa (thrombin) and factor Xa. Therefore, the cornerstone of UA/NSTEMI therapy is inhibition of thrombin and factor Xa with heparins (unfractionated or low molecular weight), fondaparinux, or bivalirudin (Table 3.12).

Unfractionated heparin

Several trials in the 1980s and 1990s demonstrated the superiority of combined therapy with intravenous **unfractionated heparin** and aspirin versus aspirin alone for preventing death

Table 3.12 ACC/AHA recommendations for anticoagulation in UA/NSTEMI

Class I

1 If an **invasive strategy** is chosen, one of four choices:
  a Enoxaparin (level of evidence A)
  b Unfractionated heparin (level of evidence A)
  c Bivalirudin (level of evidence B)
  d Fondaparinux (level of evidence B)
2 If a **conservative strategy** is chosen, one of three choices:
  a Enoxaparin (level of evidence A)
  b Unfractionated heparin (level of evidence A)
  c Fondaparinux (level of evidence B)
3 In patients in whom a conservative strategy is selected and who have an increased risk of bleeding, fondaparinux is preferable

Class IIa

For UA/NSTEMI patients in whom an initial conservative strategy is selected, enoxaparin or fondaparinux is preferable to UFH as anticoagulant therapy, unless coronary artery bypass is planned

or MI in patients with unstable coronary syndromes. A meta-analysis by Oler and colleagues demonstrated that addition of IV heparin to aspirin reduced the death or MI rate by one-third.[49] The dosing regimen of IV heparin that results in the best aPTT control and the highest safety is a 60 units/kg IV bolus, followed by a 12 units/kg/h IV infusion with standardized adjustments of infusion rate based on aPTT.[50] Measurement of aPTT is done 6 hours after starting the IV infusion of heparin, and then every 12–24 hours during the infusion, with the goal aPTT 50–70 seconds.

Enoxaparin

Low molecular weight heparin **enoxaparin** has several potential advantages over UFH for treatment of acute coronary syndromes. These include a higher anti-Xa to anti-IIa activity ratio (which results in less thrombin generation), higher bioavailability, and more predictable and potent antithrombin activity. In-hospital administration of LMWH is simpler than that of IV heparin, and frequent aPTT monitoring is not required (Table 3.13).

The strategy of LMWH with aspirin versus UFH with aspirin for treatment of UA/NSTEMI was examined in several randomized clinical trials (Table 3.14). The large ESSENCE trial

Table 3.13 Potential advantages of LMWH over UFH for treatment of UA/NSTEMI

Property	UFH	LMWH	Advantage of LMWH
Anti Xa:Anti-IIa activity	1:1	~2–3.8:1	
Plasma protein binding	Significant	Minimal	Higher bioavailability
Endothelial binding	Significant	Minimal	
Inhibition of fibrin-bound thrombin	No	Yes	
Neutralization by platelet factor 4	Significant	Minimal	Higher potency
Release of tissue factor pathway inhibitor	Minimal	Significant	
Inhibition of platelet-bound factor Xa	Minimal	Significant	
Bioavailability	~30%	90–95%	
Route of administration	IV	SC	Easier to administer
Need for aPTT monitoring	Yes	No	
Thrombocytopenia	1–2%	Rare	Safer

Table 3.14 Major trials of enoxaparin in UA/NSTEMI

Trial	Treatment	n	Major results
ESSENCE[56]	Enoxaparin vs. UFH for 2–8 days	3,171	16% relative reduction in rate of death, MI, or angina at 14 days with enoxaparin (16.6% vs. 19.8%); similar rate of major bleeding (6.5% vs. 7.0%)
TIMI 11B[57]	Enoxaparin vs. UFH for up to 14 days	3,910	Significant 17% reduction in the incidence of primary endpoint (death, MI, or urgent revascularization) with enoxaparin (12.4% vs. 14.5% with UFH)
ACUTE II[58]	Enoxaparin vs. UFH for 24–96 hours in patients receiving tirofiban	525	Similar incidence of major bleeding at 30 days; similar mortality at 30 days; less refractory ischemia and rehospitalization for unstable angina with enoxaparin (0.6% vs. 4.3% and 1.6% vs. 7.1%, respectively)

Continued

Table 3.14 Continued

Trial	Treatment	n	Major results
INTERACT[59]	Enoxaparin vs. UFH in patients receiving eptifibatide	746	Lower incidence of major bleeding at 96 hours with enoxaparin (1.8% vs. 4.6%); lower incidence of death or MI at 30 days with enoxaparin (5.0% vs. 9.0%)
AtoZ[60]	Enoxaparin vs. UFH in patients receiving tirofiban (crossover allowed from LMWH to UFH in the catheterization laboratory)	3,987	Enoxaparin noninferior to UFH in reducing death, MI, or refractory ischemia (8.4% vs. 9.4%)
SYNERGY[54]	Enoxaparin vs. UFH in patients treated with early invasive strategy	10,027	Similar rates of death or MI at 30 days (enoxaparin *noninferior* to UFH); more major bleeding (by TIMI criteria) with enoxaparin (9.1% vs. 7.6%)

demonstrated that enoxaparin was associated with less recurrent ischemic events and the need for repeat revascularization at 30 days.[51] In the TIMI 11B trial, treatment with enoxaparin resulted in a significant reduction in the composite endpoint of death, MI, or urgent target vessel revascularization, and these benefits were maintained at 1 year.[52] When the results of these two trials were pooled, there was a significant 20% reduction in death or MI at days 8, 14, and 43.[53] The rates of catheterization and PCI in these earlier trials was lower than is usually seen in current practice (e.g., only 13–17% of patients underwent PCI in ESSENCE), and these trials preceded data showing benefits of early invasive therapy in high-risk patients with ACS. Consequently, more recent investigations explored LMWH therapy in high-risk patients with UA/NSTEMI undergoing treatment with GPIIb/IIIa patients and early angiography/PCI. In particular, SYNERGY was a large trial comparing enoxaparin with UFH in patients undergoing treatment with tirofiban and early invasive therapy. The trial was designed to show the noninferiority of enoxaparin to UFH in preventing death or MI at 30 days, and enoxaparin met the noninferiority criteria at the expense of a modest increase in bleeding.[54] In a systematic review of six major trials comparing enoxaparin to unfractionated heparin in UA/NSTEMI, enoxaparin was found to be more effective in preventing death or MI, while bleeding rates were not different between the two drugs.[55] The revised 2007 AHA/ACC guidelines recommend anticoagulation with either enoxaparin or UFH when an early invasive approach is selected, whereas enoxaparin is preferred over UFH in patients treated with an initial conservative strategy (unless they are scheduled to undergo CABG within 24 hours).[2]

The usual dose of **enoxaparin** in UA/NSTEMI is 1 mg/kg subcutaneously every 12 hours. There is an option of administering an initial 30 mg *intravenous* bolus of enoxaparin, immediately followed by 1 mg/kg SC every 12 hours, which assures prompt achievement of therapeutic anti-Xa level. Otherwise, therapeutic levels of anti-Xa are achieved after two or more SC doses 12 hours apart. Use of enoxaparin is not recommended in patients with moderate or severe renal insufficiency (serum creatinine >2.5 mg/dl, creatinine clearance <30 ml/min). Morbidly obese patients (>150 kg) may have an unpredictable distribution of enoxaparin, and thus be at risk for inadequate anticoagulation. Thus, whereas routine monitoring of anti-Xa levels is not recommended in most settings, it may be desirable in special populations, such as obese patients, the elderly and those with *mild* renal insufficiency. In such cases, goal anti-Xa levels are 0.6–1.8 IU/ml.

Direct thrombin inhibitors

Direct thrombin inhibitors (DTIs) such as **hirudin, lepirudin, argatroban,** and **bivalirudin** inhibit both unbound and clotbound thrombin in a highly specific and potent manner, and do not significantly activate platelets.

Hirudin is a compound, naturally found in leech saliva. It has been studied in two large trials of patients with UA/NSTEMI, and was found to be efficacious, but to result in more bleeding than UFH.[61,62]

The large ACUITY trial[63] compared **bivalirudin** alone or with GPIIb/IIIa inhibitors to UFH or enoxaparin with GPIIb/IIIa inhibitors in patients with UA/NSTEMI. The trial demonstrated that bivalirudin alone was not inferior to UFH or enoxaparin plus GPIIb/IIIa inhibitor in terms of ischemic complications (7.8% and 7.3%, respectively), but significantly reduced the rate of major bleeding (3.0% vs. 5.7%, respectively). Addition of GPIIb/IIIa to bivalirudin anticoagulation did not significantly impact the rate of ischemic complications, but negated the advantages of bivalirudin over heparins in terms of bleeding.[63]

The REPLACE-2 trial[64] randomized 6010 patients undergoing elective or urgent PCI (including those with UA/NSTEMI) to IV bivalirudin, or the standard combination of IV unfractionated heparin and planned GPIIb/IIIa inhibitor. By 30 days after PCI, the incidence of combined endpoint of death, MI, urgent repeat revascularization, or in-hospital major bleeding was similar between the groups (9.2% vs. 10.0% for bivalirudin and UFH, respectively). When the individual components of the endpoint were analyzed, the incidence of major in-hospital bleeding was found to be significantly lower with bivalirudin (2.4% vs. 4.1%). The dose of bivalirudin used during the trial was an IV bolus of 0.75 mg/kg prior to the start of the intervention, followed by infusion of 1.75 mg/kg/h for the duration of the procedure.

On the basis of these data, the 2007 ACC/AHA guidelines recommend bivalirudin alone as an anticoagulant option in patients with UA/NSTEMI, when *invasive* strategy is employed. It is especially valuable in patients at high risk for bleeding. Provided that clopidogrel was given to the patient at least 6 hours prior to PCI, GPIIb/IIIa inhibitors may be omitted when bivalirudin is used. For patients treated with a conservative strategy, data on bivalirudin alone are lacking, and enoxaparin, UFH, or fondaparinux (see below) are preferred.[2] However, in patients with a history of **heparin-induced thrombocytopenia thrombosis syndrome (HITT)**, it is reasonable to choose bivalirudin as a single anticoagulant, even if PCI is not planned.

Fondaparinux

Fondaparinux is a synthetic pentasaccharide that selectively inhibits factor Xa, and thus causes inhibition of thrombin formation. Its advantages include once-daily subcutaneous administration, rapid and predictable absorption, and no need for frequent laboratory monitoring. Fondaparinux was initially studied in the ACS population within the small PENTUA trial, where a range of once-daily doses for 3–7 days was administered to patients treated conservatively for UA/ NSTEMI. Fondaparinux was associated with low rates of bleeding and anti-ischemic efficacy similar to enoxaparin.[65] The large OASIS-5 trial directly compared fondaparinux with enoxaparin in over 20,000 patients with ACS, with the primary outcome measure being death, nonfatal MI, or refractory ischemia at 9 days.[66] Fondaparinux was associated with a similar rate of primary endpoint compared to enoxaparin (5.8% and 5.7%, respectively); however, the rate of major bleeding at 9 days significantly favored fondaparinux (2.2% vs. 4.1% with enoxaparin). Importantly, fondaparinux was associated with a small but statistically significant increase in catheter-related thrombi (absolute increase, 0.5%). This was largely abated by using UFH at the time of PCI.

The 2007 ACC/AHA guidelines suggest that monotherapy with fondaparinux is an anticoagulant option in patients with UA/NSTEMI treated with either a conservative or an invasive strategy.[2] In the latter case, fondaparinux is usually supplemented with UFH or bivalirudin during PCI. Fondaparinux may be especially valuable in those at increased risk of bleeding.

Oral anticoagulation in UA/NSTEMI

Oral **warfarin** anticoagulation alone was shown to be superior to placebo in the treatment of myocardial infarction in the early 1990s.[67] At least ten trials compared warfarin plus aspirin with aspirin alone after ACS. The patient population spanned the entirety of the ACS spectrum. A meta-analysis of these trials demonstrated the superiority of warfarin plus aspirin versus aspirin alone in reducing the annual rate of recurrent myocardial infarction (2.2% vs. 4.1%, respectively), ischemic stroke (0.4% vs. 0.8%), and revascularization (11.5% vs. 13%). Warfarin-based strategy was associated with a statistically and clinically significant increase in major bleeding (1.5% vs. 0.6%) and overall mortality did not differ between the groups.[68]

At the present time, routine combined therapy with aspirin and warfarin is not recommended for primary treatment of UA/NSTEMI. However, oral anticoagulation with warfarin remains an important therapy for prevention of thromboembolic events in selected patients with UA/NSTEMI, including those with atrial fibrillation, severe left ventricular dysfunction, and left ventricular aneurysm. For further discussion on warfarin anticoagulation after ACS see Chapters 6 and 7.

Fibrinolysis in UA/NSTEMI

Thrombolytic therapy is **contraindicated** in patients with UA/NSTEMI. Several trials, including TIMI-IIIB, showed conclusively that thrombolytic therapy in UA/NSTEMI was associated with *more* fatal and nonfatal MI, and a higher rate of intracranial hemorrhage than heparin alone.[18] The etiology of higher ischemic event rates is incompletely elucidated, but is likely related to propagation of plaque hemorrhage by the thrombolytic, converting a partially occlusive thrombus to a complete artery occlusion.

Early lipid-lowering therapy in patients with UA/NSTEMI

Lipid-lowering therapy with an HMG-CoA reductase inhibitor (statin) should be strongly considered in all patients with UA/NSTEMI early during initial hospitalization. Long-term benefits of lipid-lowering have been well-documented in several clinical trials (for more details on secondary prevention, see Chapter 6). Recent investigations focused on early initiation of statin therapy after ACS. In the MIRACL trial,[69] 3,086 subjects with UA/NSTEMI were randomized within 24–96 hours of hospital admission to atorvastatin 80 mg daily or placebo. At 16 weeks, major adverse cardiac events (death, MI, cardiac arrest, recurrent ischemia) were reduced by 16% in the atorvastatin group (14.8% vs. 17.4% for placebo). In a large PROVE IT-TIMI 22 trial, intensive lipid-lowering therapy (atorvastatin 80 mg/d) was compared with moderate therapy (pravastatin 40 mg/d) in 4,162 patients within 10 days of an acute coronary syndrome, with or without ST-segment elevation.[70] The rate of primary endpoint (death, MI, recurrent severe angina, stroke) was reduced by 16% in the atorvastatin group, compared to the pravastatin group. Notably, median cholesterol achieved with atorvastatin 80 mg/d in PROVE IT was 62 mg/dl (1.6 mmol/l). Recently, the ARMYDA–ACS trial[71] evaluated immediate therapy with atorvastatin 80 mg/d for NSTEMI, and found a significant reduction in the rate of myocardial infarction following urgent PCI. These data should suggest starting high-dose statin *upon admission* in patients with ACS.

Patients who have sustained an acute coronary syndrome should be considered at high risk for recurrent cardiac events. ACC/AHA recommendations advocate assessment of a fasting baseline lipid profile in all patients within 24 hours of admission, and initiation of stating therapy in all patients *regardless* of baseline lipid levels and dietary modifications.[2] Based on the data above, it is reasonable to initiate intensive lipid-lowering therapy with atorvastatin 80 mg/d, or equivalent medication, with a goal LDL of <70 mg/dl. This is reflected in the latest update to the National Cholesterol Education Program Adult Treatment Panel (NCEP-ATP) III guidelines.[72]

A secondary goal of HDL > 40 mg/dl should also be achieved, by combining statins with nicotinic acid (**niacin**), or fibrates (**fenofibrate, gemfibrozil**), as further discussed in Chapter 7.

Predischarge noninvasive risk stratification after UA/NSTEMI

Exercise tolerance testing is frequently employed to diagnose or exclude ACS (primarily unstable angina) in patients with intermediate probability of having this diagnosis. In some patients with *established* UA/NSTEMI, noninvasive risk stratification is helpful prior to discharge from the hospital (Figure 3.4). Treadmill and bicycle, as well as pharmacologic stress testing with a vasodilator (e.g., adenosine or dipyridamole), is safe as early as 48 hours after presentation with a definite ACS, provided that the ECG is stable for 24 hours prior to the test, the previously elevated biomarkers of necrosis are trending down, and patient is free of anginal symptoms at rest.

Angiography ± PCI performed	Patient treated conservatively
• To assess LV systolic function and valvular disease prior to planned CABG (echo) • To assess for residual provokable ischemia in case of incomplete revascularization (exercise or pharmacologic stress testing with echo or myocardial perfusion imaging) • To assess myocardial viability and guide revascularization in a patient with multivessel disease and low LV systolic function (cardiovascular magnetic resonance imaging, radiolabeled glucose positron emission tomography, or rest-redistribution myocardial perfusion scanning) • To prescribe an exercise program for cardiac rehabilitation	• To diagnose exercise-induced ischemia and select patients for angiography ± PCI • To prescribe and exercise program for cardiac rehabilitation

Figure 3.4 Goals of noninvasive testing in patients with UA/NSTEMI.

Several modalities of noninvasive testing are available (Table 3.15). Of these, treadmill exercise tolerance testing (ETT) with either **echocardiography** or **myocardial perfusion imaging** is most commonly employed. In patients who are unable to ambulate because of pulmonary or musculoskeletal disease, pharmacologic stress testing may be employed.

Table 3.15 Noninvasive risk stratification modalities

Stress modality	Imaging method
Exercise: • Treadmill exercise • Bicycle ergometry Pharmacologic: • Dobutamine • Adenosine • Dipyridamole Pacing: • Internal • External	• ECG • Echocardiography • Single photon emission computed tomography (SPECT) myocardial perfusion scanning: ^{201}thallium, ^{99}technetium (SestaMIBI, Myoview®, Cardiolite®) • Magnetic resonance imaging • Positron emission tomography

Based on the results of the noninvasive testing, patients can generally be classified as high, moderate, and low risk for death within 1 year (Table 3.16), and the need for further revascularization can likewise be assessed.

Table 3.16 Mortality after ACS based on noninvasive testing (data from Fraker et al.[73])

High risk (>3% annual mortality)

1 LV ejection fraction <40% at rest or during exercise
2 Stress-induced large perfusion defect
3 Several stress-induced moderate perfusion defects
4 Large, fixed perfusion defect with LV cavity dilation or increased lung uptake
5 Echocardiographic evidence of stress-induced hypokinesis of >2 LV wall segments at a low dose of dobutamine, or heart rate < 120 bpm

Moderate risk (1–3% annual mortality)

1 LV ejection fraction 40–50%
2 A single stress-induced moderate perfusion defect without LV cavity dilation or increased lung uptake
3 Limited echocardiographic ischemia involving ≤2 LV wall segments at higher dobutamine doses or heart rate > 120 bpm

Low risk (<1% annual mortality)

1 Normal stress myocardial perfusion or a small stress-induced defect only
2 Normal (or unchanged from baseline) echocardiographic wall motion at stress
3 Low-risk treadmill score (≥5)

Overall management of UA/NSTEMI

As outlined in this chapter, the choice of therapies for UA/NSTEMI is largely driven by data from multiple clinical trials. Every healthcare provider taking care of a patient with UA/NSTEMI must have a clear understanding of that patient's risk profile, and must select appropriate pharmacologic and revascularization strategy, based on that profile. Risk assessment should begin immediately after presentation with symptoms of ACS, and the patient's risk should be frequently reassessed based on additional data. Use of critical pathways and checklists may facilitate adherence to the evidence-based guidelines. The overall management pathway as advocated by the 2007 ACC/AHA guidelines is given in Figures 3.1 and 3.2.

References

1. Rosamond W, Flegal K, Furie K, et al. Heart disease and stroke statistics—2008 update: a report from the American Heart

Association Statistics Committee and Stroke Statistics Subcommittee. *Circulation* 2008; 117: e25–e146.

2. Anderson JL, Adams CD, Antman EM, *et al.* ACC/AHA 2007 guidelines for the management of patients with unstable angina/ non-ST-elevation myocardial infarction: a report of the American College of Cardiology/American Heart Association Task Force on Practice Guidelines (Writing Committee to Revise the 2002 Guidelines for the Management of Patients with Unstable Angina/Non-ST-Elevation Myocardial Infarction) developed in collaboration with the American College of Emergency Physicians, the Society for Cardiovascular Angiography and Interventions, and the Society of Thoracic Surgeons endorsed by the American Association of Cardiovascular and Pulmonary Rehabilitation and the Society for Academic Emergency Medicine. *J Am Coll Cardiol* 2007; 50: e1–e157.

3. Peterson ED, Roe MT, Mulgund J, *et al.* Association between hospital process performance and outcomes among patients with acute coronary syndromes. Jama *2006*; 295: 1912–20.

4. Braunwald E. Unstable angina. A classification. *Circulation* 1989; 80: 410–4.

5. Thygesen K, Alpert JS, White HD, *et al.* Universal definition of myocardial infarction. Circulation 2007; 116: 2634–53.

6. Savonitto S, Ardissino D, Granger CB, *et al.* Prognostic value of the admission electrocardiogram in acute coronary syndromes. *Jama* 1999; 281: 707–13.

7. Antman EM, Cohen M, Bernink PJ, *et al.* The TIMI Risk Score for unstable angina/non-ST elevation MI: A method for prognostication and therapeutic decision making. *Jama* 2000; 284: 835–42.

8. Soiza RL, Leslie SJ, Williamson P, *et al.* Risk stratification in acute coronary syndromes—does the TIMI Risk Score work in unselected cases? *Qjm* 2006; 99: 81–7.

9. Sabatine MS, Morrow DA, McCabe CH, Antman EM, Gibson CM, Cannon CP. Combination of quantitative ST deviation and troponin elevation provides independent prognostic and therapeutic information in unstable angina and non-ST-elevation myocardial infarction. *Am Heart J* 2006; 151: 25–31.

10. Morrow DA, Antman EM, Snapinn SM, McCabe CH, Theroux P, Braunwald E. An integrated clinical approach to predicting the benefit of tirofiban in non-ST elevation acute coronary syndromes. Application of the TIMI Risk Score for UA/NSTEMI in PRISM-PLUS. *Eur Heart J* 2002; 23: 223–9.

11. Sabatine MS, McCabe CH, Morrow DA, *et al.* Identification of patients at high risk for death and cardiac ischemic events after hospital discharge. *Am Heart J* 2002; 143: 966–70.

12. Kini AS, Lee PC, Mitre CA, *et al*. Prediction of outcome after percutaneous coronary intervention for the acute coronary syndrome. *Am J Med* 2003; 115: 708–14.

13. The Holland Interuniversity Nifedipine/Metoprolol Trial (HINT) Research Group. Early treatment of unstable angina in the coronary care unit: a randomised, double blind, placebo controlled comparison of recurrent ischaemia in patients treated with nifedipine or metoprolol or both. *Br Heart J* 1986; 56: 400–13.

14. Gibson RS, Boden WE, Theroux P, *et al*. Diltiazem and reinfarction in patients with non-Q-wave myocardial infarction. Results of a double-blind, randomized, multicenter trial. *N Engl J Med* 1986; 315: 423–9.

15. Held PH, Yusuf S, Furberg CD. Calcium channel blockers in acute myocardial infarction and unstable angina: an overview. *Bmj* 1989; 299: 1187–92.

16. Yusuf S, Sleight P, Pogue J, Bosch J, Davies R, Dagenais G. Effects of an angiotensin-converting-enzyme inhibitor, ramipril, on cardiovascular events in high-risk patients. The Heart Outcomes Prevention Evaluation Study Investigators. *N Engl J Med* 2000; 342: 145–53.

17. Fox KM. Efficacy of perindopril in reduction of cardiovascular events among patients with stable coronary artery disease: randomised, double-blind, placebo-controlled, multicentre trial (the EUROPA study). *Lancet* 2003; 362: 782–8.

18. The TIMI IIIB Investigators. Effects of tissue plasminogen activator and a comparison of early invasive and conservative strategies in unstable angina and non-Q-wave myocardial infarction: Results of the TIMI IIIB Trial. *Circulation* 1994; 89: 1545–56.

19. Boden WE, O'Rourke RA, Crawford MH, *et al*., for the Veterans Affairs Non-Q-Wave Infarction Strategies in Hospital (VANQWISH) Trial Investigators. Outcomes in patients with acute non-Q-wave myocardial infarction randomly assigned to an invasive as compared with a conservative strategy. *N Engl J Med* 1998; 338: 1785–92.

20. McCullough PA, O'Neill WW, Graham M, *et al*. A prospective randomized trial of triage angiography in acute coronary syndromes ineligible for thrombolytic therapy. Results of the medicine versus angiography in thrombolytic exclusion (MATE) trial. *J Am Coll Cardiol* 1998; 32: 596–605.

21. FRagmin and Fast Revascularisation during InStability in Coronary artery disease Investigators. Invasive compared with non-invasive treatment in unstable coronary-artery disease: FRISC II prospective randomised multicentre study. *Lancet* 1999; 354: 708–15.

22. Spacek R, Widimsky P, Straka Z, *et al*. Value of first day angiography/angioplasty in evolving Non-ST segment elevation

myocardial infarction: an open multicenter randomized trial. The VINO Study. *Eur Heart J* 2002; 23: 230–8.

23. Cannon CP, Weintraub WS, Demopoulos LA, *et al*. Comparison of early invasive and conservative strategies in patients with unstable coronary syndromes treated with the glycoprotein IIb/IIIa inhibitor tirofiban. *N Engl J Med* 2001; 344: 1879–87.

24. Fox KA, Poole-Wilson PA, Henderson RA, *et al*. Interventional versus conservative treatment for patients with unstable angina or non-ST-elevation myocardial infarction: the British Heart Foundation RITA 3 randomised trial. Randomized Intervention Trial of unstable Angina. *Lancet* 2002; 360: 743–51.

25. Neumann FJ. Intracoronary Stenting With Antithrombotic Regimen Cooling-Off (ISAR-COOL) Study American Heart Association Scientific Sessions. Chicago, 2002.

26. de Winter RJ, Windhausen F, Cornel JH, *et al*. Early invasive versus selectively invasive management for acute coronary syndromes. *N Engl J Med* 2005; 353: 1095–104.

27. Collaborative meta-analysis of randomised trials of antiplatelet therapy for prevention of death, myocardial infarction, and stroke in high risk patients. *Bmj* 2002; 324: 71–86.

28. Topol EJ, Easton D, Harrington RA, *et al*. Randomized, double-blind, placebo-controlled, international trial of the oral IIb/IIIa antagonist lotrafiban in coronary and cerebrovascular disease. *Circulation* 2003; 108: 399–406.

29. Yusuf S, Zhao F, Mehta SR, Chrolavicius S, Tognoni G, Fox KK. Effects of clopidogrel in addition to aspirin in patients with acute coronary syndromes without ST-segment elevation. *N Engl J Med* 2001; 345: 494–502.

30. Wong JT, Nagy CS, Krinzman SJ, Maclean JA, Bloch KJ. Rapid oral challenge-desensitization for patients with aspirin-related urticaria-angioedema. *J Allergy Clin Immunol* 2000; 105: 997–1001.

31. A randomised, blinded, trial of clopidogrel versus aspirin in patients at risk of ischaemic events (CAPRIE). CAPRIE Steering Committee. *Lancet* 1996; 348: 1329–39.

32. Mehta SR, Yusuf S, Peters RJ, *et al*. Effects of pretreatment with clopidogrel and aspirin followed by long-term therapy in patients undergoing percutaneous coronary intervention: the PCI-CURE study. *Lancet* 2001; 358: 527–33.

33. Bertrand ME, Rupprecht HJ, Urban P, Gershlick AH. Double-blind study of the safety of clopidogrel with and without a loading dose in combination with aspirin compared with ticlopidine in combination with aspirin after coronary stenting: the clopidogrel aspirin stent international cooperative study (CLASSICS). *Circulation* 2000; 102: 624–9.

34. Mishkel GJ, Aguirre FV, Ligon RW, Rocha-Singh KJ, Lucore CL. Clopidogrel as adjunctive antiplatelet therapy during coronary stenting. *J Am Coll Cardiol* 1999; 34: 1884–90.
35. Wiviott SD, Braunwald E, McCabe CH, *et al*. Prasugrel versus clopidogrel in patients with acute coronary syndromes. *N Engl J Med* 2007; 357: 2001–15.
36. Bhatt DL, Topol EJ. Current role of platelet glycoprotein IIb/IIIa inhibitors in acute coronary syndromes. *Jama* 2000; 284: 1549–58.
37. Boersma E, Harrington RA, Moliterno DJ, *et al*. Platelet glycoprotein IIb/IIIa inhibitors in acute coronary syndromes: a meta-analysis of all major randomised clinical trials. *Lancet* 2002; 359: 189–98.
38. Indications for fibrinolytic therapy in suspected acute myocardial infarction: collaborative overview of early mortality and major morbidity results from all randomised trials of more than 1000 patients. Fibrinolytic Therapy Trialists' (FTT) Collaborative Group. *Lancet* 1994; 343: 311–22.
39. Platelet glycoprotein IIb/IIIa receptor blockade and low-dose heparin during percutaneous coronary revascularization. The EPILOG Investigators. *N Engl J Med* 1997; 336: 1689–96.
40. Randomised placebo-controlled and balloon-angioplasty-controlled trial to assess safety of coronary stenting with use of platelet glycoprotein-IIb/IIIa blockade. *Lancet* 1998; 352: 87–92.
41. Randomised placebo-controlled trial of abciximab before and during coronary intervention in refractory unstable angina: the CAPTURE Study. *Lancet* 1997; 349: 1429–35.
42. Simoons ML. Effect of glycoprotein IIb/IIIa receptor blocker abciximab on outcome in patients with acute coronary syndromes without early coronary revascularisation: the GUSTO IV-ACS randomised trial. *Lancet* 2001; 357: 1915–24.
43. Novel dosing regimen of eptifibatide in planned coronary stent implantation (ESPRIT): a randomised, placebo-controlled trial. *Lancet* 2000; 356: 2037–44.
44. Randomised placebo-controlled trial of effect of eptifibatide on complications of percutaneous coronary intervention: IMPACT-II. Integrilin to Minimise Platelet Aggregation and Coronary Thrombosis—II. *Lancet* 1997; 349: 1422–8.
45. Inhibition of platelet glycoprotein IIb/IIIa with eptifibatide in patients with acute coronary syndromes. The PURSUIT Trial Investigators. Platelet Glycoprotein IIb/IIIa in Unstable Angina: Receptor Suppression Using Integrilin Therapy. *N Engl J Med* 1998; 339: 436–43.

46. Effects of platelet glycoprotein IIb/IIIa blockade with tirofiban on adverse cardiac events in patients with unstable angina or acute myocardial infarction undergoing coronary angioplasty. The RESTORE Investigators. Randomized Efficacy Study of Tirofiban for Outcomes and REstenosis. *Circulation* 1997; 96: 1445–53.

47. A comparison of aspirin plus tirofiban with aspirin plus heparin for unstable angina. Platelet Receptor Inhibition in Ischemic Syndrome Management (PRISM) Study Investigators. *N Engl J Med* 1998; 338: 1498–505.

48. Inhibition of the platelet glycoprotein IIb/IIIa receptor with tirofiban in unstable angina and non-Q-wave myocardial infarction. Platelet Receptor Inhibition in Ischemic Syndrome Management in Patients Limited by Unstable Signs and Symptoms (PRISM-PLUS) Study Investigators. *N Engl J Med* 1998; 338: 1488–97.

49. Oler A, Whooley MA, Oler J, Grady D. Adding heparin to aspirin reduces the incidence of myocardial infarction and death in patients with unstable angina. A meta-analysis. *Jama* 1996; 276: 811–5.

50. Raschke RA, Reilly BM, Guidry JR, Fontana JR, Srinivas S. The weight-based heparin dosing nomogram compared with a "standard care" nomogram. A randomized controlled trial. *Ann Intern Med* 1993; 119: 874–81.

51. Cohen M, Demers C, Gurfinkel EP, *et al*. A comparison of low-molecular-weight heparin with unfractionated heparin for unstable coronary artery disease. Efficacy and Safety of Subcutaneous Enoxaparin in Non-Q-Wave Coronary Events Study Group. *N Engl J Med* 1997; 337: 447–52.

52. Antman EM, Cohen M, McCabe C, Goodman SG, Murphy SA, Braunwald E. Enoxaparin is superior to unfractionated heparin for preventing clinical events at 1-year follow-up of TIMI 11B and ESSENCE. *Eur Heart J* 2002; 23: 308–14.

53. Antman EM, Cohen M, Radley D, McCabe C, Rush J, Premmereur J, Braunwald E. Assessment of the treatment effect of enoxaparin for unstable angina/non-Q-wave myocardial infarction. TIMI 11B-ESSENCE meta-analysis. *Circulation* 1999; 100: 1602–8.

54. Ferguson JJ, Califf RM, Antman EM, *et al*. Enoxaparin vs unfractionated heparin in high-risk patients with non-ST-segment elevation acute coronary syndromes managed with an intended early invasive strategy: primary results of the SYNERGY randomized trial. *Jama* 2004; 292: 45–54.

55. Petersen JL, Mahaffey KW, Hasselblad V, *et al*. Efficacy and bleeding complications among patients randomized to enoxaparin or unfractionated heparin for antithrombin therapy in non-ST-segment elevation acute coronary syndromes: a systematic overview. *Jama* 2004; 292: 89–96.

56. Cohen M, Demers C, Gurfinkel EP, *et al.*, for the Efficacy and Safety of Subcutaneous Enoxaparin in Non-Q-Wave Coronary Events Study Group. A comparison of low-molecular-weight heparin with unfractionated heparin for unstable coronary artery disease. *N Engl J Med* 1997; 337: 447–52.

57. Antman EM, McCabe CH, Gurfinkel EP, *et al.* Enoxaparin prevents death and cardiac ischemic events in unstable angina/non-Q-wave myocardial infarction. Results of the thrombolysis in myocardial infarction (TIMI) 11B trial. *Circulation* 1999; 100: 1593–601.

58. Cohen M, Theroux P, Borzak S, *et al.* Randomized double-blind safety study of enoxaparin versus unfractionated heparin in patients with non-ST-segment elevation acute coronary syndromes treated with tirofiban and aspirin: the ACUTE II study. The Antithrombotic Combination Using Tirofiban and Enoxaparin. *Am Heart J* 2002; 144: 470–7.

59. Goodman SG, Fitchett D, Armstrong PW, Tan M, Langer A. Randomized evaluation of the safety and efficacy of enoxaparin versus unfractionated heparin in high-risk patients with non-ST-segment elevation acute coronary syndromes receiving the glycoprotein IIb/IIIa inhibitor eptifibatide. *Circulation* 2003; 107: 238–44.

60. Blazing MA, deLemos JA, White HD, *et al.* Safety and efficacy of enoxaparin vs unfractionated heparin in patients with non-ST-segment elevation acute coronary syndromes who receive tirofiban and aspirin: a randomized controlled trial. *Jama* 2004; 292: 55–64.

61. A comparison of recombinant hirudin with heparin for the treatment of acute coronary syndromes. The Global Use of Strategies to Open Occluded Coronary Arteries (GUSTO) IIb investigators. *N Engl J Med* 1996; 335: 775–82.

62. Effects of recombinant hirudin (lepirudin) compared with heparin on death, myocardial infarction, refractory angina, and revascularisation procedures in patients with acute myocardial ischaemia without ST elevation: a randomised trial. Organisation to Assess Strategies for Ischemic Syndromes (OASIS-2) Investigators. *Lancet* 1999; 353: 429–38.

63. Stone GW, McLaurin BT, Cox DA, *et al.* Bivalirudin for patients with acute coronary syndromes. *N Engl J Med* 2006; 355: 2203–16.

64. Lincoff AM, Bittl JA, Harrington RA, *et al.*, for the REPLACE-2 Investigators. Bivalirudin and Provisional Glycoprotein IIb/IIIa Blockade Compared with Heparin and Planned Glycoprotein IIb/IIIa Blockade during Percutaneous Coronary Intervention: REPLACE-2 Randomized Trial. *JAMA* 2003; 289: 853–63.

65. Simoons ML, Bobbink IW, Boland J, *et al*. A dose-finding study of fondaparinux in patients with non-ST-segment elevation acute coronary syndromes: the Pentasaccharide in Unstable Angina (PENTUA) Study. *J Am Coll Cardiol* 2004; 43: 2183–90.
66. Yusuf S, Mehta SR, Chrolavicius S, *et al*. Comparison of fondaparinux and enoxaparin in acute coronary syndromes. *N Engl J Med* 2006; 354: 1464–76.
67. Smith P, Arnesen H, Holme I. The effect of warfarin on mortality and reinfarction after myocardial infarction. *N Engl J Med* 1990; 323: 147–52.
68. Rothberg MB, Celestin C, Fiore LD, Lawler E, Cook JR. Warfarin plus aspirin after myocardial infarction or the acute coronary syndrome: meta-analysis with estimates of risk and benefit. *Ann Intern Med* 2005; 143: 241–50.
69. Schwartz GG, Olsson AG, Ezekowitz MD, *et al*. Effects of atorvastatin on early recurrent ischemic events in acute coronary syndromes: the MIRACL study: a randomized controlled trial. *Jama* 2001; 285: 1711–8.
70. Cannon CP, Braunwald E, McCabe CH, *et al*. Intensive versus moderate lipid lowering with statins after acute coronary syndromes. *N Engl J Med* 2004; 350: 1495–504.
71. Patti G, Pasceri V, Colonna G, *et al*. Atorvastatin pretreatment improves outcomes in patients with acute coronary syndromes undergoing early percutaneous coronary intervention: results of the ARMYDA–ACS randomized trial. *J Am Coll Cardiol* 2007; 49: 1272–8.
72. Grundy SM, Cleeman JI, Merz CN, *et al*. Implications of recent clinical trials for the National Cholesterol Education Program Adult Treatment Panel III guidelines. *Circulation* 2004; 110: 227–39.
73. Fraker TD, Jr., Fihn SD, Gibbons RJ, *et al*. 2007 chronic angina focused update of the ACC/AHA 2002 guidelines for the management of patients with chronic stable angina: a report of the American College of Cardiology/American Heart Association Task Force on Practice Guidelines Writing Group to develop the focused update of the 2002 guidelines for the management of patients with chronic stable angina. *J Am Coll Cardiol* 2007; 50: 2264–74.

CHAPTER 4
ST-segment-elevation myocardial infarction

Eli V. Gelfand and Christopher P. Cannon

Introduction

Acute myocardial infarction with ST-segment elevation (STEMI) accounts for approximately 30% of all presentations with ACS. Among patients with STEMI, total coronary occlusion with a thrombus is seen in >90% of cases.[1]

Diagnosis of STEMI was discussed in detail in Chapter 2. It is based upon the constellation of chest discomfort suggestive of myocardial ischemia, and an ECG with 1 mm or greater ST elevations in two or more contiguous leads or a new left bundle branch block. Depending on the timing of presentation, serum biomarkers of myocardial necrosis may or may not be elevated at the time reperfusion therapy is initiated, although some degree of myocardial necrosis is virtually inevitable.

Global treatment goals in STEMI

The latest ACC/AHA Guidelines for Management of Patients with STEMI mandate attainment of four primary goals (Table 4.1).[2] These are to be achieved promptly, and concurrently, and thus require the participation of an entire cardiovascular care team, including emergency medical technicians and paramedics, physicians, nurses, pharmacists, and radiation technologists.

Table 4.1 Primary goals for management of STEMI

1 Confirmation of the diagnosis by ECG
2 Initiation of primary reperfusion therapy
3 Relief of ischemic pain
4 Assessment of the hemodynamic state and correction of
   abnormalities that are present

Mortality in treated patients with STEMI varies greatly depending on the clinical variables at presentation. A convenient Thrombolysis in Myocardial Infarction (TIMI) Risk Score was derived based on data from the InTIME-II study (Table 4.2).[3] Application of the risk score to a population of patients with STEMI demonstrated a 20-fold gradient of increasing mortality, from 0.8 to 17.4% (Figure 4.1).

Table 4.2 The TIMI Risk Score for ST-elevation MI (from Morrow et al.[3])

Risk factor	Points
DM, history of HTN or history of angina	1
Systolic blood pressure <100 mmHg	3
Heart rate >100 bpm	2
Killip class II–IV	2
Body weight <150 lb (67 kg)	1
Anterior ST-segment elevation or left bundle branch block	1
Time to treatment > 4 hours	1
Age:	
• ≥75 years old	3
• 65–74 years old	2
• < 65 years old	0

In STEMI, the overall goal is to rapidly assess the patient's eligibility for primary reperfusion therapy, to select the type of reperfusion (i.e., pharmacological vs. mechanical), and to commence the selected therapy expeditiously.

Prehospital management and triage

Prehospital management of acute MI focuses on improving survival to hospital admission during the high-risk period in the first hour after symptom onset. The emphasis is on the

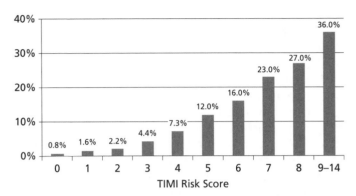

Figure 4.1 Thirty-day mortality in STEMI based on the TIMI Risk Score (data from Morrow et al.[3]).

reduction of "door-to-needle time" for patients receiving fibrinolytics, or "door-to-balloon time" for patients treated with primary percutaneous coronary intervention (PCI). This is achieved by educating the general public about the warning signs of a heart attack, by having quick-response emergency medical service (EMS) teams, by equipping populated areas with automatic external defibrillators (AED), and by training the public in their use. Unless a definite history of severe aspirin allergy is elucidated, **aspirin 162–325 mg PO, chewed** should be administered in the field to all patients suspected of having STEMI.

Prehospital fibrinolysis has been evaluated as the means to effect maximal myocardial salvage.[4] It requires a well-organized EMS system, with properly trained emergency medical personnel, and reliable physician backup. Several randomized studies compared prehospital fibrinolysis with hospital-initiated fibrinolysis or with primary PCI, and individually found no significant improvement in mortality with the prehospital strategy. A meta-analysis of six early trials, however, demonstrated a 17% reduction in all-cause in-hospital mortality with prehospital fibrinolysis.[5] Subsequently, the CAPTIM trial demonstrated a trend towards lower 30-day mortality with prehospital fibrinolysis versus primary PCI among patients randomized within 2 hours of symptom onset (2.2% vs. 5.7%).[6] This suggests that prehospital fibrinolysis within a highly selected healthcare delivery system may be a valuable treatment strategy for patients presenting *very early* after symptom onset. As such, this approach has not been widely adopted in most communities.

At this time, the ACC/AHA recommends that the prehospital fibrinolysis protocol is reasonable in settings in which physicians are present *in the ambulance*. It is also reasonable to consider prehospital fibrinolysis within a well-organized EMS system, which comprises full-time trained paramedics, 12-lead ECG systems in the field, ECG transmission capabilities, on-line medical command, a medical director with training/experience in STEMI management, and an ongoing continuous quality-improvement program.[7]

Transport decisions

The dominant reperfusion strategy for STEMI patients in the U.S. at this time is primary PCI. However, whereas virtually any U.S. hospital is capable of providing fibrinolysis, only a minority have a robust 24-hour primary PCI program. Importantly, the relative benefit of reperfusion (especially fibrinolysis) for STEMI declines rapidly. Data from the Fibrinolytic Therapy Trialists' (FTT) Collaborative Group show that the best results are achieved in patients who present within 2 hours of symptom onset.[8] If the hospital closest to the patient location has a primary PCI program, the patient should be transported there. However, the decision on whether to transport a patient with STEMI to a closer hospital *without* a PCI program, or to tolerate a longer transfer time in order to pursue primary PCI, is more complicated. Based on the comparison of fibrinolysis and primary PCI (see below), the ACC/AHA recommends that primary PCI is preferable at a *neighboring* institution if a transfer can be accomplished within 30–60 minutes.[7]

Management prior to reperfusion

Upon arrival in the emergency department of a patient with a suspected STEMI, a focused history, a targeted clinical examination, and a rapid (within 10 minutes) 12-lead ECG should be performed. Once a diagnosis of ST-elevation MI has been established, immediate treatment must be initiated. Routine measures in the ED should include the following:

- Continuous ECG monitoring.
- Frequent noninvasive blood pressure monitoring.
- Reliable intravenous access.
- Supplemental oxygen.
- Aspirin 162–325 mg, chewed (if not already administered by the emergency medical personnel).

Following this focused initial assessment and therapy, a reperfusion strategy is selected. For fibrinolysis, the goal time to initiation of IV fibrinolytic (door-to-needle time) is 30 minutes. In case of primary PCI, the goal time to inflation of angioplasty balloon in the infarct-related artery (door-to-balloon time) is 90 minutes.

Primary reperfusion therapy for STEMI

Fibrinolysis

Data from randomized controlled clinical trials involving over 50,000 patients indicate that administration of IV fibrinolytics to eligible patients with acute MI confers a 20–25% relative mortality benefit.[8] Very early administration (within 1 hour of symptom onset) results in a 6.5% absolute mortality reduction; administration 1–6 hours after symptom onset is associated with a 2–3% reduction. When administered late (>12 hours after symptom onset), fibrinolytics confer no mortality benefit.[8]

Fibrinolysis should be considered in patients who have ST-segment elevation of >1 mm (at 10 mm/mV) in two or more contiguous leads, or new left bundle branch block, in the absence of contraindications. Consideration for fibrinolysis should be given in patients who present with ≥3 mm ST segment depressions in the anterior leads. In this case, ST elevations in leads V_7–V_9 may provide a definite answer, and confirm a posterior wall MI. Because the leading adverse effect of fibrinolysis is bleeding—and, in particular, intracranial hemorrhage, which can be catastrophic—targeted assessment for contraindications to fibrinolysis is mandatory prior to initiation of therapy (Table 4.3). Use of a standard checklist may facilitate rapid and correct selection of patients appropriate for fibrinolysis (Figure 4.2).

Table 4.3 Contraindications to fibrinolytic therapy

Absolute contraindications
- Hemorrhagic stroke at any time
- Ischemic or embolic stroke within preceding 12 months
- Known intracranial neoplasm, AV malformation, or aneurysm
- Active gastrointestinal bleeding
- Suspected aortic dissection
- Trauma or major surgery within the preceding 2–4 weeks
- Pregnancy

Relative contraindications
- Blood pressure > 180/110 mmHg at presentation
- Nonhemorrhagic stroke >1 year earlier
- CPR for >10 minutes, especially with rib fractures
- Active peptic ulcer disease
- Chronic anticoagulation with warfarin

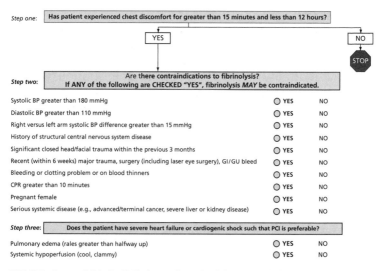

STEMI = ST-elevation myocardial infarction; BP = blood pressure; GI = gastrointestinal; GU = genitorurinary; CPR = cardiopulmonary resuscitation

Figure 4.2 A reperfusion checklist for patients with STEMI (reproduced, with permission, from Antman et al. J Am Coll Cardiol 2004; 44: 671–719[7]).

Fibrinolysis is especially underused in patients of advanced age (>75 years). While older age (especially in women) does carry with it an increased risk of bleeding complications, older patients also derive the greatest absolute mortality benefit from fibrinolysis.

Intravenous fibrinolytic agents act by activating plasminogen and promoting its conversion to plasmin. In turn, plasmin degrades fibrin and causes clot degradation. **Streptokinase (SK)** has no intrinsic enzymatic activity and must form a complex with plasminogen. In addition, both SK and **urokinase** deplete circulating fibrinogen, and thus cause a generalized, systemic lytic state. Newer agents, such as **tissue plasminogen activator (t-PA)**, **reteplase (rPA)**, and **tenecteplase (TNK)** are "fibrin-specific," and generate plasmin mostly on the surface of the existing thrombus. They deplete fibrinogen levels to a lesser degree than SK and hence have a reduced tendency to cause generalized bleeding (Table 4.4).

Table 4.4 A comparison of common fibrinolytic agents for STEMI

Agent	SK	tPA	rPA	TNK
Dose	1.5 million units over 60 minutes	15 mg bolus, then 0.75 mg/kg (maximum 50 mg) over 30 minutes, then 0.5 mg/kg (maximum 35 mg) over the next 60 minutes	10 unites over 2 minutes, then repeat 10 units at 30 minutes	Single bolus over 5–10 seconds, based on weight: <60 kg = 30 mg 60–69 kg = 35 mg 70–79 kg = 40 mg 80–89 kg = 45 mg ≥90 kg = 50 mg
Plasma half-life (minutes)	25	4–8	15	20
Fibrinogen depletion	++++	++	+++	+
90-minute patency	+	+++	++++	++++
Need for IV heparin	No	Yes	Yes	Yes

When a fibrinolytic is administered, compensatory endogenous procoagulant response is observed immediately, and is in part mediated by the rebound increase in thrombin activity.[9] Therefore *concurrent anticoagulant therapy* must be used with all fibrin-specific fibrinolytic therapies. Unfractionated heparin (UFH) administered concurrently with a fibrinolytic probably improves infarct-related artery patency, although translation into improved clinical outcomes has been less impressive.[10] The suggested regimen for UFH includes a bolus of 60 U/kg (maximum dose, 4,000 U), followed by a continuous infusion at 12 U/kg, used with tPA or rPA fibrinolysis. The goal for activated partial thromboplastin time (aPTT) should be 1.5–2.0 times control (approximately 50–70 seconds). In the ASSENT-3 trial, enoxaparin added to TNK was compared with UFH, and was associated with an improvement in recurrent ischemia and infarction.[11]

Combination fibrinolysis
Combining reduced-dose fibrinolytic with glycoprotein (GP) IIb/IIIa inhibitors has been proposed to improve infarct-related artery patency. This strategy has been tested with GPIIb/IIIa inhibitor abciximab in several prospective trials, including the large GUSTO V (with reteplase)[12] and ASSENT-3 (with tenecteplase).[11] A meta-analysis of these trials demonstrated no significant reduction in mortality with abciximab plus half-dose fibrinolytic, compared to the fibrinolytic alone.[13] There was a small decrease in reinfarction with abciximab, which was offset by an increase in major bleeding complications. Bleeding was particularly often observed in older patients. Based on these data, the ACC/AHA guidelines give this combined strategy a class IIb recommendation for prevention of recurrent infarction in selected patients—namely, those <75 years old—with anterior infarction and low risk of bleeding.[7] The regimen should not be used in older patients.

Markers of fibrinolysis effectiveness
In patients who undergo angiography following fibrinolysis, the accepted quantitative marker of artery patency is TIMI flow, which is used widely in clinical trials and commonly employed in routine interventional cardiology clinical practice (Table 4.5).[14] Fibrinolysis achieves *some* degree of patency of the infarct-related artery in approximately 80% of patients,[15] but the best outcomes are associated with normal (TIMI grade 3) flow (Figure 4.3).[15–18]

Following initiation of fibrinolytics, continuous ECG monitoring and periodic 12-lead ECGs are helpful in assessing the clinical response to therapy. Markers of effectiveness

Table 4.5 TIMI flow grade

TIMI flow grade 0	No perfusion; no antegrade flow beyond the point of occlusion
TIMI flow grade 1	Penetration without perfusion; faint antegrade coronary flow beyond the occlusion, although filling of the distal coronary bed is incomplete
TIMI flow grade 2	Delayed flow; sluggish antegrade flow with complete filling of the distal territory
TIMI flow grade 3	Complete perfusion; flow fills the distal territory completely

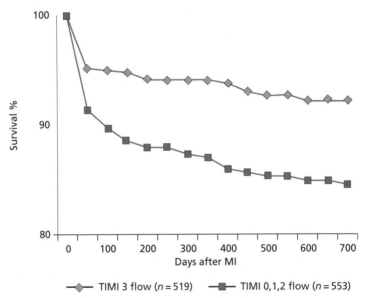

Figure 4.3 Two-year survival curves for patients enrolled in the GUSTO-1 angiographic sub-study, based on 90-minute infarct-related artery patency rates (data from Ross et al.[18]).

include a $\geq 50\%$ reduction of the initial ST-segment elevations 60–90 minutes after initiation of therapy, maintenance (or restoration) of electrical and hemodynamic stability, and relief of ischemic symptoms.[7] Accelerated idioventricular rhythm (AIVR, Chapter 6) is occasionally seen after fibrinolytic administration, and is a marker of successful reperfusion.

Worsening pain, lack of ST segment resolution 90 minutes after initiation of therapy, ventricular tachycardia or fibrillation, or sustained hemodynamic instability are all markers of unsuccessful reperfusion, and should prompt consideration for urgent transfer to a facility capable of performing rescue percutaneous or surgical revascularization.

Complications of fibrinolysis

The most common complication of fibrinolysis is bleeding at the vascular puncture sites, which is usually manageable with conservative measures. Bleeding is more commonly seen with first-generation fibrinolytics, such as SK. The primary *life-threatening* complication of fibrinolysis is intracranial hemorrhage. Emergency treatment of ICH begins with assessment of its extent using computed tomography, and cessation of fibrinolysis and all anticoagulant and antiplatelet agents. Other general measures include lowering of the intracranial pressure with head elevation and osmotic diuresis. The neurosurgical team should be consulted early, and should be ready to perform craniotomy if necessary.

Primary percutaneous coronary intervention

Primary percutaneous coronary intervention (**primary PCI**) with stent implantation should be considered the preferred reperfusion strategy for acute MI when performed by an experienced operator with available surgical backup, within 12 hours of onset of symptoms (Table 4.6). The latest developments in the techniques of coronary artery stenting, stent design, and adjunctive pharmacologic therapy during PCI have made many larger institutions rely almost exclusively on this mode of treatment for patients presenting with acute MI.

PCI can also be performed in patients who fail to achieve reperfusion with fibrinolytic therapy; this is termed **rescue PCI** and is discussed separately. Routine **PCI following fibrinolytic therapy** and **late PCI** (>12 hours following onset of symptoms) are also considered later in this chapter.

Table 4.6 ACC/AHA recommendations for primary PCI for STEMI (adapted from Antman et al.[7])

Class I

General considerations:

If immediately available, primary PCI should be performed in patients with STEMI (including true posterior MI) or MI with new LBBB who can undergo PCI of the infarct artery within 12 hours of symptom onset, if performed in a timely fashion (balloon inflation within 90 minutes of presentation) by persons skilled in the procedure (individuals who perform >75 PCI procedures per year); the procedure should be supported by experienced personnel in an appropriate laboratory environment (a laboratory that performs >200 PCI procedures per year, of which >35 are primary PCI for STEMI, and has cardiac surgery capability)

Specific considerations:

1 Primary PCI should be performed as quickly as possible, with a goal of a medical contact-to-balloon or door-to-balloon interval of within 90 minutes

2 If the symptom duration is within 3 hours and the expected door-to-balloon time minus the expected door-to-needle time is:

   a within 1 hour, primary PCI is generally preferred;

   b greater than 1 hour, fibrinolytic therapy (fibrin-specific agents) is generally preferred

3 If symptom duration is greater than 3 hours, primary PCI is generally preferred and should be performed with a medical contact-to-balloon or door-to-balloon interval as short as possible and a goal of within 90 minutes

4 Primary PCI should be performed for patients <75 years old with ST elevation or LBBB who develop shock within 36 hours of MI and are suitable for revascularization that can be performed within 18 hours of shock, unless further support is futile because of the patient's wishes or contraindications/ unsuitability for further invasive care

5 Primary PCI should be performed in patients with severe CHF and/or pulmonary edema (Killip class 3) and onset of symptoms within 12 hours; the medical contact-to-balloon or door-to-balloon time should be as short as possible (i.e., goal within 90 minutes)

Class IIa

1 Primary PCI is reasonable for selected patients ≥75 years with ST elevation or LBBB or who develop shock within 36 hours of MI and are suitable for revascularization that can be performed within 18 hours of shock; patients with good prior functional status who are suitable for revascularization and agree to invasive care may be selected for such an invasive strategy

Continued

Table 4.6 Continued

2 It is reasonable to perform primary PCI for patients with onset of symptoms
   within the prior 12–24 hours and one or more of the following:
   a severe CHF;
   b hemodynamic or electrical instability;
   c persistent ischemic symptoms

Class IIb
1 The benefit of primary PCI for STEMI patients eligible for fibrinolysis is not well
   established when performed by an operator who performs fewer than 75 PCI
   procedures per year

Class III
1 PCI should not be performed in a noninfarct artery at the time of primary PCI in
   patients without hemodynamic compromise
2 Primary PCI should not be performed in asymptomatic patients more than
   12 hours after onset of STEMI if they are hemodynamically and electrically
   stable

Comparison of PCI with fibrinolysis

The efficacy of fibrinolysis declines rapidly as time from symptom onset exceeds 2 hours (Figure 4.4), and delays in presentation frequently limit its usefulness. In parallel with expanding
PCI facilities, percutaneous revascularization (with or without
stenting) has been compared with fibrinolysis in 23 randomized trials, including 15 trials utilizing contemporary, fibrin-
specific lytic agents. Data from these trials indicate that PCI
compared with fibrinolysis results in a 25% reduction in death,
a 64% reduction in reinfarction, a 95% reduction in intracranial hemorrhage, and a 53% reduction in stroke.[19] The
primary reason for this advantage is that normal flow in the
infarct-related artery is achieved in 90–95% of patients with
primary PCI, but only 50–60% of those treated with
fibrinolysis.[16] The absolute advantage of primary PCI is greatest in high-risk patients, particularly those in cardiogenic
shock, where timely reliable revascularization is critical. The
reduction in mortality with primary PCI is likely explained by
mechanical control over an inciting ruptured plaque, resulting
in less embolization and less recurrent infarction. Successful
fibrinolysis leads to thrombus resolution, but does not

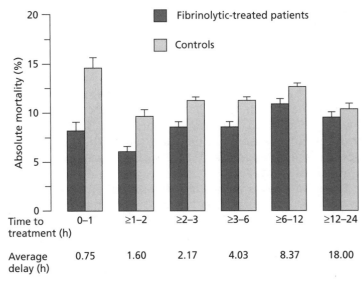

Figure 4.4 Mortality at 35 days among fibrinolytic-treated and control patients, according to time to treatment (reproduced, with permission, from Boersma et al. Lancet 1996; 348: 771–5[21]).

immediately address the ruptured plaque. Necropsy studies suggest that reperfusion injury and hemorrhagic transformation of a myocardial infarction are common following fibrinolytic therapy, but less so following mechanical revascularization.[20]

Timing of primary PCI

The latest ACC/AHA guidelines recommend achieving a door-to-balloon time of less than 90 minutes;[7] outcomes are worse with longer door-to-balloon times. Registry data demonstrate that in-hospital mortality is 41% and 62% higher in patients achieving door-to-balloon times of 121–150 minutes and 151–180 minutes, respectively, than in those who undergo PCI within 2 hours.[22] Because most hospitals in the U.S. and around the world do not have primary PCI programs, the primary question facing clinicians in these hospitals is whether to administer on-site fibrinolysis, or transfer the patient to a skilled PCI facility.

The term "PCI-related delay" is frequently used as a metric when assessing transfer times, and is defined as the difference between door-to-balloon and door-to-needle times. This parameter is useful because it accounts for hospital and transport inefficiencies, specific to the locale. For example, the local emergency transportation service may be relatively efficient in initiating inter-hospital transfer, but the hospital emergency department and pharmacy are equally prepared to commence fibrinolytic therapy within 15 minutes of the patient's arrival, and thus the PCI-related delay may be equal to that of a neighboring facility, where both facets of care are proportionally less efficient.

Several studies examined outcomes in patients transferred to skilled PCI facilities after having been initially treated at community hospitals without PCI programs. The largest trial was DANAMI-2, which was terminated prematurely after an interim analysis demonstrated significant reductions in death, reinfarction, and disabling stroke in the PCI group compared to fibrinolysis (6.7% vs. 12.3%, respectively).[23] Notably, 96% of patients were transferred for PCI in less than 2 hours. The other studies showed weaker trends towards decreased mortality with PCI. A meta-analysis combining data from all trials found a 68% reduction in the rate of reinfarction and a 56% reduction in the rate of stroke with PCI, with a trend towards a lower all-cause mortality.[24] In the context of clinical trials, transfer times between hospitals are frequently in line with the latest guidelines; however, in a "real-world" registry of acute MI, the median door-to-balloon time for transfer patients was 180 minutes, and a recommended time of <90 minutes was achieved in only 4.2% of patients.

The choice of reperfusion strategy usually depends on the availability of a nearby skilled PCI facility, transport time, and patient-specific factors (Table 4.7). A recent landmark study examined data from almost 200,000 patients at 645 hospitals, and assessed PCI-related delays, at which mortality with PCI and fibrinolysis would be equal.[25] This measure ranged greatly depending on patients' age, anatomic infarct location, and delay to hospital presentation. Indeed, for an 80-year-old patient presenting with inferior STEMI 3 hours after the onset of symptoms, even a long PCI-related delay of 179 minutes would result in equivalent outcomes between PCI

Table 4.7 The choice of reperfusion strategy in STEMI

Primary PCI preferred
- Skilled PCI laboratory with surgical backup available
  - Medicalcontact-to-balloon time <90 minutes
  - Door-to-balloontime <60 minutes
- High-risk STEMI
  - KillipClass III–IV
  - Cardiogenicshock
- Contraindications to fibrinolysis present
- Late presentation (>3 hours prior to medical contact)
- Diagnosis of STEMI is in doubt

Fibrinolysis preferred
- Early presentation (≤3 hours) and delay to PCI > 1 hour
- Lack of access to skilled PCI laboratory
- Delay to access to PCI laboratory
  - Prolonged transport
  - PCI-related delay > 1 hour
  - Medical contact-to-balloon time > 90 minutes or
    door-to-balloon time >60 minutes

---

and fibrinolysis, whereas for a 50-year-old patient with anterior STEMI less than 2 hours from symptom onset, a PCI-related delay in excess of 40 minutes would negate any mortality advantage of PCI (Figure 4.5).

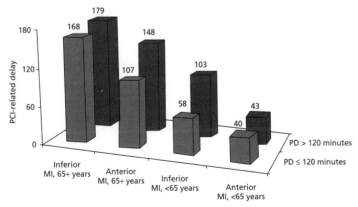

Figure 4.5 The PCI-related delay at which PCI and fibrinolysis mortality equalize (adapted, with permission, from Pinto *et al. Circulation* 2006; 114: 2019–25[25]): PD = prehospital presentation delay.

PCI following fibrinolytic therapy

Following administration of fibrinolytic therapy, PCI may be performed for three indications. **Rescue PCI** is urgent catheterization following the failure of fibrinolytic therapy to achieve clinical reperfusion of the infarct-related artery. **Facilitated PCI** is planned intervention performed after an attempt at pharmacologic reperfusion, regardless of clinical evidence of artery patency. **Delayed routine PCI** is intervention performed several days after successful fibrinolysis, irrespective of the presence of residual ischemia.

Rescue PCI

Rescue PCI was studied in five trials, including REACT[26] and MERLIN.[27] Both of these trials demonstrated that rescue PCI was associated with a significant reduction in composite endpoints of death, recurrent infarction, heart failure, and stroke.[26,27] The current guidelines for rescue PCI are listed in Table 4.8.

Facilitated PCI

Retrospective analyses of data from the PAMI and other trials indicate that restoration of blood flow in the infarct-related artery prior to PCI is associated with smaller infarct size, better LV systolic function, and improved clinical outcomes.[29,30] Therefore, it makes theoretical sense to employ the most aggressive pre-PCI strategies to restore arterial flow.

Application of full-dose fibrinolysis prior to PCI, however, has not withstood the challenge of clinical trials. Perhaps the strongest warning came from the ASSENT-4 study, which compared pretreatment with full-dose tenecteplase to placebo in the context of PCI for STEMI.[31] In this trial, facilitated PCI performed *within 2 hours following fibrinolysis* compared with standard primary PCI was associated with a significant 39% increase in the primary endpoint of the composite of death, heart failure, or shock within 90 days (19% vs. 13%). Indeed, each endpoint was worse with facilitated PCI, including significantly higher rates of strokes (1.8% vs. 0%, respectively), reinfarction (6% vs. 4%, respectively) and target vessel

Table 4.8 ACC/AHA guidelines for invasive strategy following fibrinolytic therapy (from Antman et al.[28])

Class I

A strategy of coronary angiography with intent to perform PCI (or emergency CABG) is recommended for patients who have received fibrinolytic therapy and have any of the following:

a cardiogenic shock in patients less than 75 years who are suitable candidates for revascularization;

b severe congestive heart failure and/or pulmonary edema (Killip class III);

c hemodynamically compromising ventricular arrhythmias

Class IIa

1 A strategy of coronary angiography with intent to perform PCI (or emergency CABG) is reasonable in patients 75 years of age or older who have received fibrinolytic therapy, and are in cardiogenic shock, provided that they are suitable candidates for revascularization

2 It is reasonable to perform rescue PCI for patients with one or more of the following:

a hemodynamic or electrical instability;

b persistent ischemic symptoms

A strategy of coronary angiography with intent to perform rescue PCI is reasonable for patients in whom fibrinolytic therapy has failed (ST-segment elevation less than 50% resolved after 90 minutes following initiation of fibrinolytic therapy in the lead showing the worst initial elevation) and a moderate or large area of myocardium at risk (anterior MI, inferior MI with right ventricular involvement, or precordial ST-segment depression)

Class IIb

A strategy of coronary angiography with intent to perform PCI in the absence of one or more of the above Class I or IIa indications might be reasonable in moderate- and high-risk patients, but its benefits and risks are not well established; the benefits of rescue PCI are greater the earlier it is initiated after the onset of ischemic discomfort

Class III

A strategy of coronary angiography with intent to perform PCI (or emergency CABG) is not recommended in patients who have received fibrinolytic therapy if further invasive management is contraindicated or the patient or designee does not wish further invasive care

revascularization (7% vs. 3%) within 90 days. Most of the strokes in the tenecteplase group were hemorrhagic.[31] Therefore, the planned strategy of full-dose lytic followed by PCI within 1–3 hours should be avoided.

A combination of reduced-dose fibrinolytics and IIb/IIIa inhibitors improves artery reperfusion, and IIb/IIIa inhibitors improve outcomes in patients undergoing primary PCI. Despite an initial enthusiasm for this strategy, several adequately powered trials demonstrated no decrease in the rate of ischemic complications with this combination therapy[32,33], and therefore such a strategy is also not recommended.

Routine PCI after successful fibrinolysis

Most patients in the U.S. treated with fibrinolytic therapy eventually undergo PCI during their index hospitalization.[34] Previously discussed data suggest that lytic therapy restores normal TIMI 3 flow in <70% of infarct-related arteries, and more reliable results can be ultimately achieved with PCI. In contrast, with facilitated PCI performed within 2 hours of lytic therapy, delaying PCI by 3 hours to several days improves outcomes, while mostly avoiding the worrisome increase in bleeding complications.[35,36] In the TRANSFER-AMI trial,[37] patients with STEMI who presented to centers where timely primary PCI was not feasible were randomized to a pharmacoinvasive strategy, consisting of emergency transfer for PCI within 6 hours of fibrinolysis or to standard treatment after fibrinolysis (transfer for *rescue* PCI only). The incidence of primary endpoint of death, MI, heart failure, severe recurrent ischemia, or shock was 10.5% in the pharmacoinvasive arm versus 16.5% in the standard treatment arm. Pharmacoinvasive strategy was associated with a significantly lower rate of recurrent infarction (3.3% vs. 6.0%) and recurrent ischemia (0.2% vs. 2.2%), indicating that such strategy, employed in a 6-hour treatment window, is efficacious.[37] A similar approach was used in the CARESS trial[38], where STEMI patients admitted to community hospitals were initially treated with heparin, half-dose reteplase, and abciximab, and were then randomized to pharmacoinvasive therapy or standard therapy with rescue PCI if needed. In the end, 86% of the immediate PCI group versus 30% of the standard care group actually received PCI. Death, MI, or refractory ischemia at 30 days was significantly reduced in the pharmacoinvasive group compared with standard care (4.4% vs. 10.7%), with most of the benefit driven by a substantial reduction in refractory ischemia (0.3% vs. 4.0%).[38]

The latest update to the ACC/AHA guidelines predates both TRANSFER-AMI and CARESS trials, and suggests that it is reasonable to perform PCI following fibrinolysis in high-risk patients, defined as those with LVEF ≤40 %, ventricular arrhythmias, or heart failure during the acute episode (Table 4.8).[28] The guidelines recognize that late PCI of a *totally occluded* infarct-related artery in stable patients with single- or two-vessel disease is not indicated or recommended.

Overall reperfusion strategy

Data presented earlier demonstrate that the choice of reperfusion strategy in STEMI is driven by hospital capabilities, geographic proximity to skilled PCI facilities, time between symptom onset and presentation, and the patient's risk profile. One suggested algorithm for strategy selection is presented in Figure 4.6.

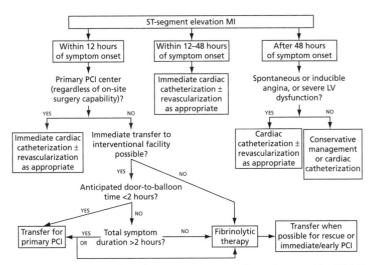

Figure 4.6 An algorithm for management of patients with STEMI (adapted, with permission, from Stone *Circulation* 2008; 118: 552–66[39]).

Coronary artery bypass grafting for treatment of STEMI

With increasing success of primary PCI techniques, emergency CABG for evolving STEMI has taken a supporting role. The 2004 ACC/AHA guidelines recommend emergency CABG in patients with acute MI who have persistent or recurrent ischemia refractory to medical therapy, who have coronary anatomy suitable for surgery, and who are not candidates for PCI.[40] Bypass grafting can be safely performed at any time following acute MI[41], although the guidelines advocate delaying surgery for several days in stable patients to allow for a degree of myocardial healing.

Adjunctive pharmacologic treatment of STEMI

Antiplatelet agents

Aspirin

In absence of a true aspirin allergy, all patients with STEMI should receive this medication as soon as the diagnosis is considered, regardless of whether the patient is a candidate for reperfusion with fibrinolysis, or primary PCI. An initial dose of 162–325 mg chewed should be given, and a subsequent daily dose of 75–100 mg is then recommended indefinitely. In the ISIS-2 trial, treatment of acute MI with aspirin 160 mg/day for 30 days resulted in a significant 23% reduction in 5-week vascular mortality (2.4 cardiovascular deaths prevented for every 100 patients treated).[42] This was equivalent to the treatment effect of streptokinase in the same trial. When aspirin was added to fibrinolysis with streptokinase, the 5-week cardiovascular mortality was reduced by 42%. In a more recent meta-analysis of antiplatelet therapy in 15 trials of acute MI, treatment with aspirin was associated with a 30% reduction in one-month mortality, and an absolute benefit of 3.8 cardiovascular events prevented for every 100 patients treated.[43] For patients with aspirin allergy, clopidogrel should be given (see below) and subsequent aspirin desensitization strongly considered. One commonly utilized desensitization protocol is suggested in the Appendix.

Clopidogrel

Dual antiplatelet therapy with aspirin and clopidogrel following fibrinolysis was studied in the CLARITY-TIMI 28 and COMMIT/CCS-2 trials.[44,45] In CLARITY-TIMI 28, patients <75 years old undergoing fibrinolysis were treated with aspirin and randomized to clopidogrel (300 mg loading dose, followed by 75 mg daily), or placebo. All patients underwent angiography 2–8 days following fibrinolysis to assess coronary patency. Clopidogrel was associated with a reduction in the primary primary endpoint of TIMI grade 0/1 flow on angiography, or death/recurrent MI if no angiography (15.0% vs. 21.7% for placebo). Bleeding was similar between the groups.[44] In COMMIT/CCS-2, patients with a suspected acute MI were randomized to clopidogrel 75 mg daily or placebo, on the background of aspirin therapy. Fibrinolytic therapy was given to one-half of the patients. Sixteen days following initiation of therapy, mortality was significantly lower in the clopidogrel group compared to placebo (7.5% vs. 8.1%, respectively), as was death, MI, or stroke.[45]

Clopidogrel in addition to aspirin is also routinely given to patients undergoing **primary PCI**. Although formal randomized trial data for this approach are lacking, extrapolation of NSTEACS trial results gives it credibility. Pretreatment with a 600 mg loading dose of clopidogrel may reduce thrombotic complications during PCI and improve outcomes, although this has not been formally tested in a randomized trial involving STEMI patients.[46]

Pretreatment with clopidogrel results in increased incidence of bleeding after coronary artery bypass grafting.[47] Therefore, for patients in whom primary PCI is planned, some centers prefer to give clopidogrel *in the catheterization laboratory*, after the coronary anatomy has been delineated, and it has been determined that immediate CABG is not needed. Overall guidelines for clopidogrel use in STEMI are outlined in Table 4.9.

Prasugrel

The novel thienopyridine prasugrel (discussed in more detail in Chapter 3) is likely to play an important role in STEMI management. In the TRITON-TIMI 38 trial, about 3,000 patients had STEMI. Compared with clopidgorel, prasugrel

Table 4.9 ACC/AHA guidelines for clopidogrel use in STEMI (from Antman et al.[28])

Class I

1 Clopidogrel 75 mg per day orally should be added to aspirin in patients with STEMI regardless of whether they undergo reperfusion with fibrinolytic therapy or do not receive reperfusion therapy; treatment with clopidogrel should continue for at least 14 days

2 In patients taking clopidogrel in whom CABG is planned, the drug should be withheld for at least 5 days and preferably for 7 days unless the urgency for revascularization outweighs the risks of excess bleeding

Class IIa

1 In patients less than 75 years of age who receive fibrinolytic therapy or who do not receive reperfusion therapy, it is reasonable to administer an oral loading dose of clopidogrel 300 mg (no data are available to guide decision-making regarding an oral loading dose in patients 75 years of age or older)

2 Long-term maintenance therapy (e.g., 1 year) with clopidogrel (75 mg per day orally) is reasonable in STEMI patients regardless of whether they undergo reperfusion with fibrinolytic therapy or do not receive reperfusion therapy

was associated with a lower risk of cardiovascular death, nonfatal MI, or nonfatal stroke, but no increase in bleeding.[48] The incidence of stent thrombosis was reduced by 50% in the prasugrel group.

Glycoprotein IIb/IIIa inhibitors
The use of GPIIb/IIIa inhibitors in combination with fibrinolytic therapy was previously discussed (see "Combination fibrinolysis").

In the catheterization laboratory during primary PCI
Intravenous GP IIb/IIIa inhibitors **abciximab, tirofiban**, and **eptifibatide** have their main use in ST-elevation MI as part of the adjunctive treatment *at the time of primary PCI*. The largest trial evaluating GPIIb/IIIa for this indication was CADILLAC,[49] where administration of abciximab in the catheterization laboratory to patients undergoing primary PCI reduced the rates of subacute thrombosis (1% with stenting alone, 0% with stenting plus abciximab) and the need for target vessel revascularization by 6 months

(8.3% and 5.2%, respectively). There was no difference in mortality between stenting alone and stenting plus abciximab.

In the emergency department prior to PCI
Recent data suggest that routine pretreatment of patients with GPIIb/IIIa inhibitors as part of the facilitated PCI strategy may improve coronary flow and ST segment resolution,[50] but does not significantly affect the efficacy of primary PCI.[51,52]

Anticoagulation therapy
A summary of the updated ACC/AHA guidelines on adjunctive anticoagulation therapy is presented in Table 4.10.

Table 4.10 ACC/AHA guidelines on adjunctive anticoagulation therapy (adapted from Antman *et al.*[28])

Class I

1 Patients undergoing reperfusion with fibrinolytics should receive anticoagulant therapy for a minimum of 48 hours and preferably for the duration of the index hospitalization, up to 8 days (regimens other than UFH are recommended if anticoagulant therapy is given for more than 48 hours because of the risk of heparin-induced thrombocytopenia with prolonged UFH treatment).

2 Anticoagulant regimens with established efficacy include the following:

  a **UFH** (initial intravenous bolus 60 U/kg [maximum 4,000 U]) followed by an intravenous infusion of 12 U/kg/h (maximum 1,000 U/h) initially, adjusted to maintain the activated partial thromboplastin time at 1.5–2.0 times control (50–70 seconds).

  b **Enoxaparin** (provided that the serum creatinine is <2.5 mg/dl in men and <2.0 mg/dl in women): for patients <75 years of age, an initial 30 mg IV bolus is given, followed 15 minutes later by subcutaneous injections of 1.0 mg/kg every 12 hours; for patients ≥75 years of age, the initial intravenous bolus is eliminated and the subcutaneous dose is reduced to 0.75 mg per kg every 12 hours. Regardless of age, if the creatinine clearance (using the Cockroft–Gault formula) during the course of treatment is estimated to be <30 ml per minute, the subcutaneous regimen is 1.0 mg/kg every 24 hours. Maintenance dosing with enoxaparin should be continued for the duration of the index hospitalization, up to 8 days.

  c **Fondaparinux** (provided that the serum creatinine is <3.0 mg per dl): initial dose 2.5 mg intravenously; subsequently subcutaneous injections of 2.5 mg once daily. Maintenance dosing with fondaparinux should be continued for the duration of the index hospitalization, up to 8 days.

Continued

Table 4.10 Continued

3 For patients undergoing PCI after having received an anticoagulant regimen, the following dosing recommendations should be followed:

  a For prior treatment with UFH, administer additional boluses of UFH as needed to support the procedure, taking into account whether GP IIb/IIIa receptor antagonists have been administered. Bivalirudin may also be used in patients treated previously with UFH.

  b For prior treatment with enoxaparin, if the last subcutaneous dose was administered within the prior 8 hours, no additional enoxaparin should be given; if the last subcutaneous dose was administered at least 8–12 hours earlier, an intravenous dose of 0.3 mg/kg of enoxaparin should be given.

  c For prior treatment with fondaparinux, administer additional intravenous treatment with an anticoagulant possessing anti-IIa activity, taking into account whether GP IIb/IIIa receptor antagonists have been administered.

Class III

1 Because of the risk of catheter thrombosis, fondaparinux should not be used as the sole anticoagulant to support PCI. An additional anticoagulant with anti-IIa activity should be administered.

Unfractionated heparin

There are limited randomized data on the benefit of **unfractionated heparin (UFH)** in acute MI. Heparin appears important in attenuating the compensatory thrombin activity **following fibrinolysis**, and thus its use is routine in patients undergoing fibrinolysis with fibrin-specific agents (Table 4.10). Routine bolus dose of UFH in this situation should be 60 U/kg IV, and should not exceed 4,000 U. This is followed by 12 U/kg/h IV infusion, not to exceed 1,000 U/h. After an uncomplicated PCI, there is rarely a need to continue UFH, whereas in the case of fibrinolysis, IV UFH is continued for 48 hours, with a goal PTT of 1.5–2.0 times control (approximately 50–70 seconds). Intravenous heparin is routinely given to patients undergoing primary PCI, because reduces acute vessel closure.[53] Activated clotting time (ACT; goal of 250–350 seconds) is used to guide heparin dosing during PCI, with IV boluses given to reach that goal.

Enoxaparin

Low molecular weight heparin **enoxaparin** is at least as safe and effective as UFH in treatment of acute MI. In the

ASSENT-3 trial,[11] treatment with enoxaparin and TNK was associated with fewer major ischemic events than UFH and TNK, with similar rates of bleeding. In the ENTIRE-TIMI 23 trial,[54] patients treated with enoxaparin and TNK had a lower 30-day rate of mortality and recurrent MI, as compared to UFH and TNK (4.4% vs. 15.9%, respectively). In the EXTRACT-TIMI 25 trial, patients with STEMI were treated with fibrinolysis and randomized to enoxaparin for the duration of hospitalization or UFH for at least 48 hours. Enoxaparin therapy was associated with a 17% reduction in the risk of death or MI at 30 days (9.9% vs. 12% for UFH).[55] Again, more bleeding was observed in the enoxaparin group (2.1% vs. 1.4%). A recent meta-analysis comparing enoxaparin to UFH in STEMI patients treated with fibrinolysis concluded that while enoxaparin was associated with higher rates of bleeding, this was substantially offset by a reduction in death and MI; for every 1,000 patients treated with enoxaparin, four major bleeds are caused, but 21 deaths or MIs are prevented.[56]

In most patients, enoxaparin 30 mg IV bolus, followed by 1 mg/kg subcutaneously every 12 hours, could be used when TNK is given. In patients >75 years of age, the IV bolus should be avoided, as it is associated with excess ICH, compared with UFH.[57]

Bivalirudin
Experience with the direct thrombin inhibitor **bivalirudin** is more limited than that with UFH or enoxaparin. The HERO-2 trial found that when added to streptokinase fibrinolysis, bivalirudin was comparable with UFH in terms of 30-day mortality (10.8% and 10.9%, respectively), but was associated with a 30% decrease in recurrent infarction compared with UFH, at the expense of a small absolute increase in mild or moderate bleeding.[58] Because wider data in patients treated with fibrinolytics are not available, the ACC/AHA guidelines limit bivalirudin use to patients with known history of heparin-induced thrombocytopenia, as an alternative to heparin.

Data for bivalirudin use in primary PCI come from the recent HORIZONS-AMI trial, in which patients were randomized to treatment with heparin plus a GPIIb/IIIa inhibitor or to treatment with bivalirudin alone.[59] Bivalirudin monotherapy was associated with lower 30-day rate of net adverse clinical events, specified as combination of bleeding, death, reinfarction, target-vessel revascularization for ischemia, and stroke (9.2% vs. 12.1% for heparin + GPIIb/IIIa). This reduction was primarily driven by a lower rate of major bleeding with bivalirudin (4.9% vs. 8.3%, respectively). The most recent guidelines preceded HORIZONS-AMI trial and thus do not endorse bivalirudin use in primary PCI; this is likely to evolve.

Fondaparinux
Synthetic factor Xa inhibitor **fondaparinux** was systematically studied in the large OASIS-6 trial.[60] Of the enrolled STEMI patients, slightly under one-half did not have a strict indication for heparin (e.g., streptokinase use). In this group, fondaparinux 2.5 mg/day for 8 days or until hospital discharge was compared to placebo as adjunctive therapy, mostly to streptokinase fibrinolysis. Fondaparinux was associated with a significant reduction in death or recurrent MI (11.2% vs. 14.0% for placebo). In the rest of the patients, heparin was indicated for various indications, most common being invasive strategy with primary PCI, rescue PCI, or fibrinolytic therapy with fibrin-specific agents. In this group, fondaparinux 2.5 mg/day for 8 days or until discharge was also compared with placebo, on top of primary reperfusion therapy. In this group, no significant reduction in death or recurrent MI with fondaparinux was seen (8.3% vs. 8.7% for heparin). In addition, among patients treated with primary PCI, an increase in guiding catheter thrombosis and intraprocedural coronary complications was seen.[60] Thus, one should avoid fondaparinux use during primary PCI. Fondaparinux should be used with streptokinase.

Warfarin
Warfarin is not routinely used as adjunctive therapy in STEMI. When given to patients with acute MI either alone (goal INR, 2.8–4.2), or in combination with aspirin (goal INR, 2.0–2.5), it reduces the incidence of death, recurrent

infarction and stroke, as compared to aspirin alone.[61] This is achieved at the expense of the higher risk of bleeding. These benefits are in the range of what is seen with clopidogrel, for which monitoring is less intensive, and outcome data are more robust. Therefore, current recommendations for warfarin after an acute MI are limited to the following situations:

- Ejection fraction less than 30% with or without heart failure.
- Atrial fibrillation (indefinite anticoagulation).
- Left ventricular thrombus or aneurysm.

Other adjunctive therapy

Beta adrenergic blockers
Recent trial data brought renewed controversy to routine aggressive use of beta-blockers in acute STEMI. Earlier guidelines advocated early intravenous beta-blockade in patients with acute MI. The large COMMIT/CCS2 trial systematically examined beta-blockade in STEMI by randomizing >45,000 patients within 24 hours of onset of suspected MI to receive up to three doses of metoprolol 5 mg IV in the first 15 minutes, followed by 200 mg orally daily or matching placebo.[62] Metoprolol reduced the risk of reinfarction and ventricular fibrillation (absolute reduction of 0.5% for each), but did not significantly impact in-hospital mortality. Importantly, in patients with evidence of left ventricular systolic dysfunction or heart failure on admission, intravenous metoprolol was associated with a significant increase in the risk of cardiogenic shock (absolute increase of 1.1%).[62] The latest update to the ACC/AHA guidelines was therefore updated to include these data, and suggests using IV beta-blockade only in patients who are hypertensive and without evidence of heart failure or LV dysfunction (Table 4.11).

Inhibitors of the renin–angiotensive–aldosterone axis

Angiotensin-converting enzyme inhibitors and angiotensin receptor blockers
Angiotensin-converting enzyme (ACE) inhibitors attenuate left ventricular remodeling following acute STEMI, inhibit

Table 4.11 ACC/AHA guidelines for beta-blockers in STEMI (adapted from Antman et al.[28])

Class I

1 **Oral beta-blocker therapy** should be initiated in the first 24 hours for patients who do not have any of the following:
   a signs of heart failure
   b evidence of a low output state
   c increased risk for cardiogenic shock
   d other relative contraindications to beta-blockade—
      i PR interval greater than 240 ms
      ii second- or third-degree heart block
      iii active asthma, or reactive airway disease
2 Patients with early contraindications within the first 24 hours of STEMI should be reevaluated for candidacy for beta-blocker therapy as secondary prevention.

Class IIa

It is reasonable to administer an **IV beta-blocker** at the time of presentation to STEMI patients who are **hypertensive** and who do not have any of the following:
a signs of heart failure:
b evidence of a low output state
c increased risk for cardiogenic shock
d other relative contraindications to beta-blockade—
   i PR interval greater than 240 ms
   ii second- or third-degree heart block
   iii active asthma, or reactive airway disease

Class III

Intravenous beta-blockers should not be administered to STEMI patients who have any of the following:
a signs of heart failure
b evidence of a low output state
c increased risk for cardiogenic shock
d other relative contraindications to beta-blockade—
   i PR interval greater than 240 ms
   ii second- or third-degree heart block
   iii active asthma, or reactive airway disease

LV dilation, and promote recovery of LV systolic function.[63] Early administration appears to be more effective than later therapy.[64] Current recommendations from ACC/AHA suggest that ACE inhibitors should be started in all high-risk patients with STEMI (Table 4.12). Features signifying high risk include anterior infarction, clinical heart failure, or ejection fraction

Table **4.12** ACC/AHA guidelines for inhibition of the renin–angiotensin–aldosterone axis in STEMI (adapted from Antman *et al.*[7])

Class I

1 An ACE inhibitor should be administered orally within the first 24 hours of STEMI to patients with anterior infarction, pulmonary congestion, or LVEF <40%, in the absence of hypotension (systolic blood pressure <100 mmHg or <30 mmHg below baseline) or known contraindications to that class of medications.

2 An angiotensin receptor blocker (ARB) should be administered to STEMI patients who are intolerant of ACE inhibitors and who have either clinical or radiological signs of heart failure, or LVEF < 40%. Valsartan and candesartan have established efficacy for this recommendation.

Class IIa

An ACE inhibitor administered orally within the first 24 hours of STEMI can be useful in patients without anterior infarction, pulmonary congestion, or LVEF <40% in the absence of hypotension (systolic blood pressure < 100 mmHg or < 30 mmHg below baseline) or known contraindications to that class of medications. The expected treatment benefit in such patients is less (5 lives saved per 1,000 patients treated) than for patients with LV dysfunction.

Class III

An intravenous ACE inhibitor should not be given to patients within the first 24 hours of STEMI because of the risk of hypotension. (A possible exception may be patients with refractory hypertension.)

<40%. A systematic overview of data from 100,000 patients, treated with ACE-I early (0–36 hours) after an acute MI, demonstrated a 7% proportional reduction in mortality by 30 days, with most benefit occurring in the first week. This indicates that ACE-I therapy for acute MI should be started preferably in the first 24 hours after the index event.[65] In the same overview, while the absolute mortality benefit was greatest in the high-risk population of those with anterior MI, Killip class II–III or tachycardia on presentation, the proportional benefit was similar in patients with different underlying risk. Since then, large HOPE and EUROPA trials have demonstrated that in a broad population of subjects *at risk* for cardiovascular disease, but without known heart failure or low ejection fraction, ACE-I significantly reduced the incidence of death, myocardial infarction, and stroke.[66,67]

Together, these data support initiation of an ACE inhibitor in most patients with an acute MI, provided that hypotension is avoided. Data behind long-term use of ACE inhibitors in patients with CAD is well-established, and discussed in Chapter 7.

Angiotensin receptor blockers (ARBs) are equivalent, but not superior to ACE inhibitors in the setting of acute MI.[68,69] The VALIANT trial demonstrated that combination therapy with ARB and AVE inhibitors is associated with excess side effects, including clinically significant hypotension.[69] The primary role of ARBs in the acute setting at this time is in ACE inhibitor-intolerant patients (Table 4.12).

Aldosterone receptor blockers
The EPHESUS trial shed light on utility of eplerenone in the setting of acute MI.[70] Patients who sustained an acute MI 3–14 days earlier and had either diabetes mellitus or clinical evidence of heart failure were randomized to eplerenone or placebo. Eplerenone therapy was associated with a 15% reduction in all-cause mortality and a 17% reduction in cardiovascular death or hospitalization for cardiovascular events compared with placebo. A 21% relative risk reduction in sudden cardiac death was observed. Eplerenone was associated with a significantly increased risk of serious hyperkalemia (5.5% vs. 3.9% for placebo).[70] The updated ACC/AHA guidelines recommend mirror the inclusion criteria for EPHESUS trial, including a serum creatinine cutoff of 2.5 mg/dl, and emphasize the importance of monitoring renal function and serum potassium during ongoing therapy with an aldosterone receptor blocker.

Nitrates
Nitroglycerin (NTG) therapy is useful in treating ischemic pain during acute MI. Whereas studies in the pre-fibrinolysis era demonstrated mortality reduction with nitrates, more recent trials showed neutral effects on mortality, when NTG is used alongside reperfusion. Initial dosing should be sublingual (0.4 mg SL every 5 minutes until pain is relieved, or a maximum of three doses). If pain does not subside after sublingual NTG, intravenous infusion could be started (20–200 mcg/min). Care should be taken to avoid hypotension. Nitroglycerin therapy is contraindicated in the presence of

right ventricular infarction, where it can precipitate hypotension by reducing ventricular preload (see Chapter 6).

Calcium channel blockers

Calcium channel blockers (CCB) have a very limited role in treating patients with STEMI, as no CCB has ever been conclusively demonstrated to improve outcomes in acute MI. Specifically, short-acting nifedipine should be avoided, as it can precipitate substantial reflex tachycardia. Verapamil or diltiazem may infrequently be used for relief of ongoing ischemia when beta-blockers are ineffective or contraindicated for the relief of ongoing ischemia. The same two agents can occasionally be useful for rate control of rapid atrial fibrillation complicating acute MI. Because of the negative inotropic and chronotropic effects of nondihydropyridine CCBs, these drugs should not be used in patients with heart failure, LV dysfunction, or atrioventricular block.[28]

Analgesics and anxiolytics

Acute MI is almost invariably associated with at least moderate discomfort, which can contribute to hypertension, tachycardia, and worsening ischemia. Morphine possesses strong analgetic properties, and is both a potent venodilator, and a mild arterial dilator. Thus, it reduces ventricular preload and decreases myocardial oxygen demand, making it an ideal choice for pain relief in STEMI. Morphine sulfate (2–4 mg IV with increments of 2–8 mg IV repeated at 5- to 15-minute intervals) is typically effective and safe. In presence of hypovolemia, or right ventricular MI, morphine can cause significant hypotension. The usual care must also be taken to avoid excessive sedation and respiratory depression.

Significant anxiety is seen in many patients around the time of myocardial infarction. It is often especially notable in relatively young patients with the first diagnosis of MI, and is frequently accompanied by insomnia. Use of anxiolytic medications can improve sleep, and may hasten recovery in such patients. Typical agents used are benzodiazepines, such as oxazepam, diazepam, and lorazepam.

Antiarrhythmic agents

Clinically significant ventricular arrhythmias are observed in approximately 10% of STEMI patients; most occur in the first 48 hours following reperfusion.[71] Judicious use of beta-blockers in hemodynamically stable patients reduces the incidence of ventricular fibrillation.[62] Serum electrolytes should be monitored and maintained in the normal range, with serum potassium level > 4.0 mEq/l and serum magnesium > 2.0 mEq/l. Formerly a cornerstone of acute MI management, routine antiarrhythmic therapy is no longer used in stable patients following successful reperfusion of acute STEMI.

Any significant increase in ventricular irritability, or the presence of sustained ventricular arrhythmia, should prompt a search for recurrent ischemia/infarction. For further discussion on management of ventricular tachyarrhythmia following acute MI, see Chapter 6.

Treatment of hyperglycemia

Hyperglycemia during acute MI is associated with higher risk of death, cardiogenic shock, or congestive heart failure, regardless of whether the patient has previously known diabetes (see Chapter 5).[72] Mismatch of the necessary substrate and energy during ischemia-induced switch to anaerobic metabolism may underlie these detrimental effects. Maintenance of tight metabolic control during an acute MI with intravenous insulin and glucose during was tested in the DIGAMI study.[73] In that trial, hyperglycemic patients treated with 24 hours of IV insulin, followed by 3 months of SC insulin had a 29% mortality reduction at 1 year, compared to those treated with conventional therapy. Mortality reduction was most pronounced (52%) in patients with no prior insulin therapy, and in those with a low cardiovascular risk profile. The guidelines given Class I recommendation to starting an intravenous insulin infusion to normalize blood glucose (80–100 mg/dl) in critically ill patients with STEMI, and class IIa recommendation for same therapy even in patients with an uncomplicated course.[7]

Hospital care following successful reperfusion

General care

Most patients with acute STEMI are admitted to a coronary care unit (CCU), where continuous telemetry monitoring and rapid access to defibrillation is essential. Selected low-risk patients—young, with inferior STEMI, single-vessel disease and hemodynamic stability—may be managed in stepdown units following successful reperfusion. Patients initially admitted to the CCU may be transferred to the stepdown units after 12–24 hours of stability.

Continuous nasal oxygen administration is routine in the acute phase of STEMI, but in the absence of hypoxemia several hours after reperfusion, it may be stopped.

Prolonged bed rest is discouraged in patients with acute MI,[74] as it predisposes to orthostasis and syncope during initial ambulation, and is associated with lung atelectasis and venous thromboembolism. Thus, 12–18 hours after successful reperfusion, patients should be encouraged to routinely sit in a bedside armchair, and to have bedside commode privileges. Patients may begin to ambulate 24 hours after acute MI, with nursing supervision.

Hospitalization for acute MI presents a unique opportunity for the clinical team to educate the patient about lifestyle and risk factor modification, necessary to prevent recurrent vascular events. In addition, new and ongoing medications should be reviewed with the patient in detail by the treating team. Table 4.13 provides a recommended structure for educating patients after their myocardial infarction.

Table 4.13 Milestones and recommended information for educating the patient with ST-elevation myocardial infarction (adapted, with permission, from Antman *et al. J Am Coll Cardiol* 2004; 44: 671–719[7])

Before the event (ongoing by primary care provider, especially with high-risk patients):
- Assess and manage cardiac risk factors
- Review recommendations for recognizing and responding to heart attack symptoms (see http://www.nhlbi.nih.gov/health/prof/heart/mi/provider.htm)

On the day of admission (in the emergency department):
- Explain diagnosis
- Review plan for inpatient treatment and projected length of stay

Inpatient testing/procedures (day of admission until discharge):
- Explain the purpose of tests and procedures that are ordered
- Describe what to expect with tests and procedures: duration; level of discomfort and invasiveness; sensory information

---

Continued

Table 4.13 Continued

On the day of admission (in the CCU/stepdown unit):
- Orient to surroundings/routine of unit
- Explain the nursing care plan
- Describe the importance of reporting symptoms and needs

At discharge:
- Review risk factor goals and management plan
- Review prescribed medications and lifestyle changes/recommendations
- Review information on recognizing and responding to heart attack symptoms
- Recommend that family member(s) attend a CPR training program and cardiac support group
- Refer patient to cardiac rehabilitation program
- Schedule a follow-up appointment with the primary care provider
- Discuss plans for obtaining prescribed medication that day (immediately after discharge)

At follow-up visits with primary care provider (first follow-up appointment and ongoing):
- Review diagnosis with patient and hospital course/outcome
- Review medical and lifestyle regimens prescribed
- Ensure aggressive risk factor modification and follow-up
- Discuss recognition and response to acute symptoms; review action plan, including taking nitroglycerin in response to acute symptoms if prescribed, and calling 9-1-1
- Assess for depression and other psychosocial responses

Noninvasive risk stratification after STEMI

Estimation of left ventricular systolic function

Timely delivery of effective primary reperfusion therapy for STEMI is the most important predictor of in-hospital mortality, but clearly does not ensure that recurrent vascular events do not occur after discharge. One of the most robust predictors of long-term prognosis is LV ejection fraction (LVEF). Patients with reduced LVEF are at a higher risk of mortality and heart failure.[75,76] Therefore, measurement of LVEF prior to discharge is recommended in all patients with STEMI. Because LV systolic function often improves in the first 2–3 weeks following acute MI, clinicians should understand that this "acute LVEF" may overestimate the degree and extent of regional myocardial dysfunction in the long term.

Assessment of LVEF is most commonly done using transthoracic echocardiography, although radionuclide ventriculography can also be used. Cardiovascular magnetic resonance (CMR) is the gold standard for assessment of LV volumes, mass, and function, and offers an ability to quantitatively assess the infarct extent. Data are emerging about the power of CMR to predict the risk of post-MI mortality beyond information offered by LVEF alone.[77]

Stress testing
Prior to widespread use of primary PCI, stress testing prior to discharge was routine practice. Currently, inpatient stress testing is not mandatory in patients who undergo complete revascularization with PCI, but should still be performed in the outpatient setting, prior to initiating cardiac rehabilitation.

In patients who undergo incomplete revascularization (e.g., PCI to single infarct-related artery on a background of multivessel disease), stress testing is useful to detect significant residual ischemia. In sufficiently low risk patients (Table 4.14), stress testing is very safe.

Table 4.14 Safety assessment of STEMI patients prior to stress testing

1 No heart failure or recurrent angina
2 Stable ECG for 48–72 hours prior to the exercise test
3 No life-threatening cardiac arrhythmias
4 Patient underwent in-hospital cardiac rehabilitation/physical therapy assessment
5 Sufficient time has elapsed since hospital presentation:
   a 3–5 days for submaximal testing (modified Bruce or Naugton protocol);
   b >5 days for symptom-limited testing

Timing of hospital discharge following STEMI
Hospital stays after acute MI have declined steadily, from 3–4 weeks in the 1950s to several days currently. Even more recently, between 1986 and 1999, the average length of stay in a regional group of hospitals fell by 50%, from 12 to 6 days, without an effect on short-term mortality.[78] Today, low-risk patients with nonanterior STEMI, complete revascularization, normal or mildly depressed LVEF, and no post-infarct angina may be discharged on hospital day 2–3. Patients with anterior MI may be discharged on hospital

day 4–5 in the absence of complications. Close outpatient follow-up with the patient's primary care doctor and a cardiologist should be arranged, and the patient should be educated about their diagnosis as outlined in Table 4.13.

References

1. DeWood MA, Spores J, Notske R, et al. Prevalence of total coronary occlusion during the early hours of transmural myocardial infarction. N Engl J Med 1980; 303: 897–902.
2. Antman EM, Anbe DT, Armstrong PW, et al. ACC/AHA guidelines for the management of patients with ST-elevation myocardial infarction; A report of the American College of Cardiology/American Heart Association Task Force on Practice Guidelines (Committee to Revise the 1999 Guidelines for the Management of patients with acute myocardial infarction). J Am Coll Cardiol 2004; 44: E1–E211.
3. Morrow DA, Antman EM, Giugliano RP, et al. A simple risk index for rapid initial triage of patients with ST-elevation myocardial infarction: an InTIME II substudy. Lancet 2001; 358: 1571–5.
4. Milavetz JJ, Giebel DW, Christian TF, Schwartz RS, Holmes DR, Jr., Gibbons RJ. Time to therapy and salvage in myocardial infarction. J Am Coll Cardiol 1998; 31: 1246–51.
5. Morrison LJ, Verbeek PR, McDonald AC, Sawadsky BV, Cook DJ. Mortality and prehospital thrombolysis for acute myocardial infarction: A meta-analysis. Jama 2000; 283: 2686–92.
6. Steg PG, Bonnefoy E, Chabaud S, et al. Impact of time to treatment on mortality after prehospital fibrinolysis or primary angioplasty: data from the CAPTIM randomized clinical trial. Circulation 2003; 108: 2851–6.
7. Antman EM, Anbe DT, Armstrong PW, et al. ACC/AHA guidelines for the management of patients with ST-elevation myocardial infarction—executive summary. A report of the American College of Cardiology/American Heart Association Task Force on Practice Guidelines (Writing Committee to revise the 1999 guidelines for the management of patients with acute myocardial infarction). J Am Coll Cardiol 2004; 44: 671–719.
8. Indications for fibrinolytic therapy in suspected acute myocardial infarction: collaborative overview of early mortality and major morbidity results from all randomised trials of more than 1000 patients. Fibrinolytic Therapy Trialists' (FTT) Collaborative Group. Lancet 1994; 343: 311–22.
9. Eisenberg PR. Role of heparin in coronary thrombolysis. Chest 1992; 101: 131S–139S.

10. de Bono DP, Simoons ML, Tijssen J, et al. Effect of early intravenous heparin on coronary patency, infarct size, and bleeding complications after alteplase thrombolysis: results of a randomised double blind European Cooperative Study Group trial. Br Heart J 1992; 67: 122–8.

11. Efficacy and safety of tenecteplase in combination with enoxaparin, abciximab, or unfractionated heparin: the ASSENT-3 randomised trial in acute myocardial infarction. Lancet 2001; 358: 605–13.

12. Topol EJ. Reperfusion therapy for acute myocardial infarction with fibrinolytic therapy or combination reduced fibrinolytic therapy and platelet glycoprotein IIb/IIIa inhibition: the GUSTO V randomised trial. Lancet 2001; 357: 1905–14.

13. De Luca G, Suryapranata H, Stone GW, et al. Abciximab as adjunctive therapy to reperfusion in acute ST-segment elevation myocardial infarction: a meta-analysis of randomized trials. Jama 2005; 293: 1759–65.

14. Chesebro JH, Knatterud G, Roberts R, et al. Thrombolysis in Myocardial Infarction (TIMI) Trial, Phase I: A comparison between intravenous tissue plasminogen activator and intravenous streptokinase. Clinical findings through hospital discharge. Circulation 1987; 76: 142–54.

15. An international randomized trial comparing four thrombolytic strategies for acute myocardial infarction. The GUSTO investigators. N Engl J Med 1993; 329: 673–82.

16. The effects of tissue plasminogen activator, streptokinase, or both on coronary-artery patency, ventricular function, and survival after acute myocardial infarction. The GUSTO Angiographic Investigators. N Engl J Med 1993; 329: 1615–22.

17. Karagounis L, Sorensen SG, Menlove RL, Moreno F, Anderson JL. Does thrombolysis in myocardial infarction (TIMI) perfusion grade 2 represent a mostly patent artery or a mostly occluded artery? Enzymatic and electrocardiographic evidence from the TEAM-2 study. Second Multicenter Thrombolysis Trial of Eminase in Acute Myocardial Infarction. J Am Coll Cardiol 1992; 19: 1–10.

18. Ross AM, Coyne KS, Moreyra E, et al. Extended mortality benefit of early postinfarction reperfusion. GUSTO-I Angiographic Investigators. Global Utilization of Streptokinase and Tissue Plasminogen Activator for Occluded Coronary Arteries Trial. Circulation 1998; 97: 1549–56.

19. Keeley EC, Boura JA, Grines CL. Primary angioplasty versus intravenous thrombolytic therapy for acute myocardial infarction: a quantitative review of 23 randomised trials. Lancet 2003; 361: 13–20.

20. Waller BF, Rothbaum DA, Pinkerton CA, et al. Status of the myocardium and infarct-related coronary artery in 19 necropsy patients with acute recanalization using pharmacologic (streptokinase, r-tissue plasminogen activator), mechanical

(percutaneous transluminal coronary angioplasty) or combined types of reperfusion therapy. *J Am Coll Cardiol* 1987; 9: 785–801.

21. Boersma E, Maas AC, Deckers JW, Simoons ML. Early thrombolytic treatment in acute myocardial infarction: reappraisal of the golden hour. *Lancet* 1996; 348: 771–5.

22. Cannon CP, Gibson CM, Lambrew CT, *et al*. Relationship of symptom-onset-to-balloon time and door-to-balloon time with mortality in patients undergoing angioplasty for acute myocardial infarction. *Jama* 2000; 283: 2941–7.

23. Andersen HR, Nielsen TT, Rasmussen K, *et al*. A comparison of coronary angioplasty with fibrinolytic therapy in acute myocardial infarction. *N Engl J Med* 2003; 349: 733–42.

24. Dalby M, Bouzamondo A, Lechat P, Montalescot G. Transfer for primary angioplasty versus immediate thrombolysis in acute myocardial infarction: a meta-analysis. *Circulation* 2003; 108: 1809–14.

25. Pinto DS, Kirtane AJ, Nallamothu BK, *et al*. Hospital delays in reperfusion for ST-elevation myocardial infarction: implications when selecting a reperfusion strategy. *Circulation* 2006; 114: 2019–25.

26. Gershlick AH, Stephens-Lloyd A, Hughes S, *et al*. Rescue angioplasty after failed thrombolytic therapy for acute myocardial infarction. *N Engl J Med* 2005; 353: 2758–68.

27. Sutton AG, Campbell PG, Graham R, *et al*. A randomized trial of rescue angioplasty versus a conservative approach for failed fibrinolysis in ST-segment elevation myocardial infarction: the Middlesbrough Early Revascularization to Limit INfarction (MERLIN) trial. *J Am Coll Cardiol* 2004; 44: 287–96.

28. Antman EM, Hand M, Armstrong PW, *et al*. 2007 focused update of the ACC/AHA 2004 guidelines for the management of patients with ST-elevation myocardial infarction: a report of the American College of Cardiology/American Heart Association Task Force on Practice Guidelines. *J Am Coll Cardiol* 2008; 51: 210–47.

29. Brodie BR, Stuckey TD, Hansen C, Muncy D. Benefit of coronary reperfusion before intervention on outcomes after primary angioplasty for acute myocardial infarction. *Am J Cardiol* 2000; 85: 13–18.

30. Stone GW, Cox D, Garcia E, *et al*. Normal flow (TIMI-3) before mechanical reperfusion therapy is an independent determinant of survival in acute myocardial infarction: analysis from the primary angioplasty in myocardial infarction trials. *Circulation* 2001; 104: 636–41.

31. Primary versus tenecteplase-facilitated percutaneous coronary intervention in patients with ST-segment elevation acute

myocardial infarction (ASSENT-4 PCI): randomised trial. *Lancet* 2006; 367: 569–78.

32. Kastrati A, Mehilli J, Schlotterbeck K, *et al.* Early administration of reteplase plus abciximab vs abciximab alone in patients with acute myocardial infarction referred for percutaneous coronary intervention: a randomized controlled trial. *Jama* 2004; 291: 947–54.

33. Ellis SG, Tendera M, de Belder MA, *et al.* Facilitated PCI in patients with ST-elevation myocardial infarction. *N Engl J Med* 2008; 358: 2205–17.

34. Spencer FA, Goldberg RJ, Frederick PD, Malmgren J, Becker RC, Gore JM. Age and the utilization of cardiac catheterization following uncomplicated first acute myocardial infarction treated with thrombolytic therapy (The Second National Registry of Myocardial Infarction [NRMI-2]). *Am J Cardiol* 2001; 88: 107–11.

35. Fernandez-Aviles F, Alonso JJ, Pena G, *et al.* Primary angioplasty vs. early routine post-fibrinolysis angioplasty for acute myocardial infarction with ST-segment elevation: the GRACIA-2 non-inferiority, randomized, controlled trial. *Eur Heart J* 2007; 28: 949–60.

36. Fernandez-Aviles F, Alonso JJ, Castro-Beiras A, *et al.* Routine invasive strategy within 24 hours of thrombolysis versus ischaemia-guided conservative approach for acute myocardial infarction with ST-segment elevation (GRACIA-1): a randomised controlled trial. *Lancet* 2004; 364: 1045–53.

37. Cantor W. Trial of Routine ANgioplasty and Stenting After Fibrinolysis to Enhance Reperfusion in Acute Myocardial Infarction (TRANSFER-AMI). *Presented at the American College of Cardiology 2008 Scientic Sessions/i2 Summit-SCAI Annual Meeting; March 30, 2008; Chicago, IL.*

38. Di Mario C, Dudek D, Piscione F, *et al.* Immediate angioplasty versus standard therapy with rescue angioplasty after thrombolysis in the Combined Abciximab REteplase Stent Study in Acute Myocardial Infarction (CARESS-in-AMI): an open, prospective, randomised, multicentre trial. *Lancet* 2008; 371: 559–68.

39. Stone GW. Angioplasty strategies in ST-segment-elevation myocardial infarction: part II: intervention after fibrinolytic therapy, integrated treatment recommendations, and future directions. *Circulation* 2008; 118: 552–66.

40. Eagle KA, Guyton RA, Davidoff R, *et al.* ACC/AHA 2004 guideline update for coronary artery bypass graft surgery: a report of the American College of Cardiology/American Heart Association Task Force on Practice Guidelines (Committee to Update the 1999 Guidelines for Coronary Artery Bypass Graft Surgery). *Circulation* 2004; 110: e340–e437.

41. Lee JH, Murrell HK, Strony J, *et al*. Risk analysis of coronary bypass surgery after acute myocardial infarction. *Surgery* 1997; 122: 675–80; discussion 680–1.
42. Randomised trial of intravenous streptokinase, oral aspirin, both, or neither among 17,187 cases of suspected acute myocardial infarction: ISIS-2. ISIS-2 (Second International Study of Infarct Survival) Collaborative Group. *Lancet* 1988; 2: 349–60.
43. Collaborative meta-analysis of randomised trials of antiplatelet therapy for prevention of death, myocardial infarction, and stroke in high risk patients. *Bmj* 2002; 324: 71–86.
44. Sabatine MS, Cannon CP, Gibson CM, *et al*. Addition of clopidogrel to aspirin and fibrinolytic therapy for myocardial infarction with ST-segment elevation. *N Engl J Med* 2005; 352: 1179–89.
45. Chen ZM, Jiang LX, Chen YP, *et al*. Addition of clopidogrel to aspirin in 45,852 patients with acute myocardial infarction: randomised placebo-controlled trial. *Lancet* 2005; 366: 1607–21.
46. Cuisset T, Frere C, Quilici J, *et al*. Benefit of a 600-mg loading dose of clopidogrel on platelet reactivity and clinical outcomes in patients with non-ST-segment elevation acute coronary syndrome undergoing coronary stenting. *J Am Coll Cardiol* 2006; 48: 1339–45.
47. Yende S, Wunderink RG. Effect of clopidogrel on bleeding after coronary artery bypass surgery. *Crit Care Med* 2001; 29: 2271–5.
48. Wiviott SD, Braunwald E, McCabe CH, *et al*. Prasugrel versus clopidogrel in patients with acute coronary syndromes. *N Engl J Med* 2007; 357: 2001–15.
49. Stone GW, Grines CL, Cox DA, *et al*. Comparison of angioplasty with stenting, with or without abciximab, in acute myocardial infarction. *N Engl J Med* 2002; 346: 957–66.
50. Van't Hof AW, Ten Berg J, Heestermans T, *et al*. Prehospital initiation of tirofiban in patients with ST-elevation myocardial infarction undergoing primary angioplasty (On-TIME 2): a multicentre, double-blind, randomised controlled trial. *Lancet* 2008; 372: 537–46.
51. Keeley EC, Boura JA, Grines CL. Comparison of primary and facilitated percutaneous coronary interventions for ST-elevation myocardial infarction: quantitative review of randomised trials. *Lancet* 2006; 367: 579–88.
52. Ellis SG. The Facilitated Intervention with Enhanced Reperfusion Speed to Stop Events (FINESSE) trial. *Presented at the European Society of Cardiology Annual Congress, Vienna, September 1–5, 2007.*
53. Popma JJ, Berger P, Ohman EM, Harrington RA, Grines C, Weitz JI. Antithrombotic therapy during percutaneous coronary intervention: the Seventh ACCP Conference on Antithrombotic and Thrombolytic Therapy. *Chest* 2004; 126: 576S–599S.

54. Antman EM, Louwerenburg HW, Baars HF, et al. Enoxaparin as adjunctive antithrombin therapy for ST-elevation myocardial infarction: results of the ENTIRE-Thrombolysis in Myocardial Infarction (TIMI) 23 Trial. *Circulation* 2002; 105: 1642–9.

55. Antman EM, Morrow DA, McCabe CH, et al. Enoxaparin versus unfractionated heparin with fibrinolysis for ST-elevation myocardial infarction. *N Engl J Med* 2006; 354: 1477–88.

56. Murphy SA, Gibson CM, Morrow DA, et al. Efficacy and safety of the low-molecular weight heparin enoxaparin compared with unfractionated heparin across the acute coronary syndrome spectrum: a meta-analysis. *Eur Heart J* 2007; 28: 2077–86.

57. Wallentin L, Goldstein P, Armstrong PW, et al. Efficacy and safety of tenecteplase in combination with the low-molecular-weight heparin enoxaparin or unfractionated heparin in the prehospital setting: the Assessment of the Safety and Efficacy of a New Thrombolytic Regimen (ASSENT)-3 PLUS randomized trial in acute myocardial infarction. *Circulation* 2003; 108: 135–42.

58. White H. Thrombin-specific anticoagulation with bivalirudin versus heparin in patients receiving fibrinolytic therapy for acute myocardial infarction: the HERO-2 randomised trial. *Lancet* 2001; 358: 1855–63.

59. Stone GW, Witzenbichler B, Guagliumi G, et al. Bivalirudin during primary PCI in acute myocardial infarction. *N Engl J Med* 2008; 358: 2218–30.

60. Yusuf S, Mehta SR, Chrolavicius S, et al. Effects of fondaparinux on mortality and reinfarction in patients with acute ST-segment elevation myocardial infarction: the OASIS-6 randomized trial. *Jama* 2006; 295: 1519–30.

61. Hurlen M, Abdelnoor M, Smith P, Erikssen J, Arnesen H. Warfarin, aspirin, or both after myocardial infarction. *N Engl J Med* 2002; 347: 969–74.

62. Chen ZM, Pan HC, Chen YP, et al. Early intravenous then oral metoprolol in 45,852 patients with acute myocardial infarction: randomised placebo-controlled trial. *Lancet* 2005; 366: 1622–32.

63. Pfeffer MA, Lamas GA, Vaughan DE, Parisi AF, Braunwald E. Effect of captopril on progressive ventricular dilatation after anterior myocardial infarction. *N Engl J Med* 1988; 319: 80–6.

64. Pfeffer MA, Greaves SC, Arnold JM, et al. Early versus delayed angiotensin-converting enzyme inhibition therapy in acute myocardial infarction. The healing and early afterload reducing therapy trial. *Circulation* 1997; 95: 2643–51.

65. Indications for ACE inhibitors in the early treatment of acute myocardial infarction: systematic overview of individual data

from 100,000 patients in randomized trials. ACE Inhibitor Myocardial Infarction Collaborative Group. *Circulation* 1998; 97: 2202–12.

66. Yusuf S, Sleight P, Pogue J, Bosch J, Davies R, Dagenais G. Effects of an angiotensin-converting-enzyme inhibitor, ramipril, on cardiovascular events in high-risk patients. The Heart Outcomes Prevention Evaluation Study Investigators. *N Engl J Med* 2000; 342: 145–53.

67. Fox KM. Efficacy of perindopril in reduction of cardiovascular events among patients with stable coronary artery disease: randomised, double-blind, placebo-controlled, multicentre trial (the EUROPA study). *Lancet* 2003; 362: 782–8.

68. Dickstein K, Kjekshus J. Effects of losartan and captopril on mortality and morbidity in high-risk patients after acute myocardial infarction: the OPTIMAAL randomised trial. Optimal Trial in Myocardial Infarction with Angiotensin II Antagonist Losartan. *Lancet* 2002; 360: 752–60.

69. Pfeffer MA, McMurray JJ, Velazquez EJ, *et al*. Valsartan, captopril, or both in myocardial infarction complicated by heart failure, left ventricular dysfunction, or both. *N Engl J Med* 2003; 349: 1893–906.

70. Pitt B, Remme W, Zannad F, *et al*. Eplerenone, a selective aldosterone blocker, in patients with left ventricular dysfunction after myocardial infarction. *N Engl J Med* 2003; 348: 1309–21.

71. Newby KH, Thompson T, Stebbins A, Topol EJ, Califf RM, Natale A. Sustained ventricular arrhythmias in patients receiving thrombolytic therapy: incidence and outcomes. The GUSTO Investigators. *Circulation* 1998; 98: 2567–73.

72. Capes SE, Hunt D, Malmberg K, Gerstein HC. Stress hyperglycaemia and increased risk of death after myocardial infarction in patients with and without diabetes: a systematic overview. *Lancet* 2000; 355: 773–8.

73. Malmberg K, Ryden L, Efendic S, *et al*. Randomized trial of insulin-glucose infusion followed by subcutaneous insulin treatment in diabetic patients with acute myocardial infarction (DIGAMI study): effects on mortality at 1 year. *J Am Coll Cardiol* 1995; 26: 57–65.

74. Mitchell AM, Dealy JB, Lown B, Levine SA. Further observations on the armchair treatment of acute myocardial infarction. *J Am Med Assoc* 1954; 155: 810–4.

75. Burns RJ, Gibbons RJ, Yi Q, *et al*. The relationships of left ventricular ejection fraction, end-systolic volume index and infarct size to six-month mortality after hospital discharge following myocardial infarction treated by thrombolysis. *J Am Coll Cardiol* 2002; 39: 30–6.

76. Nicolosi GL, Latini R, Marino P, *et al*. The prognostic value of predischarge quantitative two-dimensional echocardiographic measurements and the effects of early lisinopril treatment on left

ventricular structure and function after acute myocardial infarction in the GISSI-3 Trial. Gruppo Italiano per lo Studio della Sopravvivenza nell'Infarto Miocardico. *Eur Heart J* 1996; 17: 1646–56.

77. Yan AT, Shayne AJ, Brown KA, *et al*. Characterization of the peri-infarct zone by contrast-enhanced cardiac magnetic resonance imaging is a powerful predictor of post-myocardial infarction mortality. *Circulation* 2006; 114: 32–9.

78. Spencer FA, Lessard D, Gore JM, Yarzebski J, Goldberg RJ. Declining length of hospital stay for acute myocardial infarction and postdischarge outcomes: a community-wide perspective. *Arch Intern Med* 2004; 164: 733–40.

CHAPTER 5
Special considerations in acute coronary syndromes

Jason Ryan and Eli V. Gelfand

Secondary unstable angina

A number of conditions alter the myocardial supply/demand relationship through mechanisms other than arterial obstruction and may also result in myocardial ischemia (Table 5.1). It is important to note that presence of one of these conditions does not preclude the possibility of concomitant obstructive coronary disease. Thus, any patient with symptoms of angina should be evaluated for obstructive coronary disease before the syndrome is considered secondary to an unrelated condition.

Acute coronary syndrome in patients with diabetes mellitus

General considerations

Patients with diabetes are at increased risk for coronary artery disease in general, and ACS in particular. A frequently cited population-based study from Finland compared 1,373 nondiabetics to 1,059 diabetics and found that the 7-year risk of myocardial infarction for diabetics *without* a history of CAD was similar to that of nondiabetics *with* a history of CAD (20% vs. 19%; Figure 5.1), making diabetes a "coronary disease equivalent."[1] The 7-year rates of death from CAD were also similar for these groups, and these similarities

Management of Acute Coronary Syndromes   Eli V. Gelfand and Christopher P. Cannon
© 2009 John Wiley & Sons, Ltd

Table 5.1 Representative causes of secondary unstable angina/myocardial infarction

Condition	Mechanism of ischemia	Goals of therapy
Severe aortic stenosis	• ↑ LV mass → ↑ O_2 demand • Compression of intramyocardial coronary arteries • Impaired myocardial relaxation • Tachycardia in the setting of "fixed" cardiac output • ↓ Coronary flow reserve	Aortic valve replacement (percutaneous balloon valvuloplasty if AVR not feasible)
Severe anemia	• ↓ O_2 delivery	Transfusion
Hypotension	• ↓ Myocardial tissue perfusion	Correction of underlying cause of hypotension; avoidance of pure vasoconstrictors during treatment
Tachycardia	• ↓ Diastolic coronary perfusion	Treat arrhythmia itself; treat underlying cause of sinus tachycardia
Fever	• ↑ Myocardial metabolic demand • ↓ Diastolic coronary perfusion	Treat underlying cause of fever
Thyrotoxicosis	• Coronary vasospasm • ↓ Diastolic coronary perfusion	Treat hyperthyroidism

persisted during long-term follow-up.[2] In addition to higher risk of developing ACS, diabetics have worse outcomes compared to nondiabetics.[3,4] Adverse events are more frequent, including arrhythmia, cardiogenic shock, heart failure, renal failure, and death. At angiography, diabetics are more likely to have left main or three-vessel coronary disease.[5]

Primary ACS therapy in diabetics
The treatment for ACS in patients with diabetes is similar to that for nondiabetics. Medical therapies including aspirin, beta-blockers, ACE inhibitors, statins, and IIB/IIIA inhibitors have been shown to have similar or greater impact on outcomes among diabetics compared to nondiabetics. Primary PCI and thrombolysis for STEMI also have similar or greater

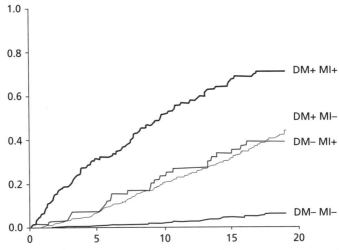

Figure 5.1 Coronary heart disease mortality over 18 years in a Finnish population with diabetes and prior myocardial infarction (adapted, with permission, from Juutilainen *et al. Diabetes Care* 2005; 28: 2901–7[2]): DM = diabetes mellitus; MI = myocardial infarction.

efficacy among diabetics. Older literature suggested that beta-blockers should be avoided in diabetics due to concerns of masking hypoglycemic episodes through blockade of the sympathetic nervous system. In recent years, however, many trials have shown definitive benefit for beta-blockers following ACS in diabetic patients. Patients must be advised that beta-blockers at high doses may mask symptoms of hypoglycemia, which should provide further motivation for close blood glucose monitoring in this population.

Glycemic control in diabetics with ACS
There is some evidence that tighter glycemic control among diabetics with ACS improves outcomes. The DIGAMI trial randomized 620 diabetic patients with STEMI to routine care or intensive therapy with intravenous insulin infusion, and found that intensive therapy reduced long-term mortality.[6] However, more recent studies have not confirmed this benefit.[7,8] The ACC/AHA guidelines for STEMI give a class I recommendation to insulin use to normalize blood glucose in patients with a complicated course, regardless of whether they have

Table 5.2 Sample insulin sliding scale for diabetics with ACS

Glucose	Insulin dose
0–50 mg/dl	4 oz. juice
51–150 mg/dl	0 units
151–200 mg/dl	2 units
201–250 mg/dl	4 units
251–300 mg/dl	6 units
301–350 mg/dl	8 units
351–400 mg/dl	10 units
>400 mg/dl	Notify M.D.

diabetes.[9] A class IIa recommendation was given to use of an insulin infusion in all other patients with MI with hyperglycemia. Table 5.2 illustrates sample insulin orders for an ACS patient based on blood glucose levels.

Coronary revascularization in diabetics
A special area of consideration for diabetics with ACS is revascularization with coronary artery bypass surgery (CABG). For patients with STEMI, CABG is usually not an option for primary therapy given the need for rapid revascularization, which can be more easily accomplished with thrombolytics or primary PCI. However, among diabetics undergoing angiography post-thrombolysis or for UA or NSTEMI, careful consideration must be given to the choice between stenting or CABG.

In the BARI trial comparing balloon angioplasty to CABG in patients with two- or three-vessel disease, diabetics had improved survival with CABG.[10] Subgroup analysis demonstrated that the benefit of CABG in diabetics was limited to those receiving an internal mammary artery bypass graft. In the ARTS I trial comparing bare-metal stenting to bypass surgery, diabetics had worse event-free survival at one year with stenting compared to CABG.[11] This difference was driven by the higher need for revascularization due to in-stent restenosis following PCI. A more recent CARDIa trial utilized PCI with drug-eluting stents, and suggested that diabetic patients with multi-vessel disease or complex single-vessel disease, but not left main disease, have a similar incidence of death, MI, or stroke at 12 months with either PCI or CABG.[12]

However, if PCI was chosen as an initial strategy, then a higher incidence of repeat revascularization was seen. On the other hand, there were more strokes in the CABG arm. The SYNTAX trial used revascularization with paclitaxel-eluting stents and compared that strategy with CABG in patients with left main and/or three-vessel disease.[13] In a subgroup analysis of patients with diabetes, there was a significantly lower 1-year incidence of major adverse cardiovascular events with CABG compared to with PCI (14.2% vs. 26.0%).

Based on these data, CABG is still the preferred revascularization strategy for diabetics with left main and/or three-vessel coronary disease, even if a predominantly drug-eluting stent-based PCI strategy is employed.

Metabolic syndrome and ACS

The metabolic syndrome (MetS) is a cluster of disorders known to promote atherosclerosis and increase cardiovascular risk. The Adult Treatment Panel III (ATP III)[14] report has defined five criteria for MetS:

1 Abdominal obesity (waist > 40 inches for men, 35 inches for women).
2 Elevated triglycerides ($\geq$150 mg/dl).
3 Low HDL cholesterol (<40 mg/dl for men, <50 mg/dl for women).
4 Elevated blood pressure ($\geq$130/$\geq$85 mmHg).
5 Elevated fasting glucose ($\geq$110 mg/dl).

The reported incidence of MetS following ACS is high, ranging from 29 to 46%. MetS is particularly prevalent among those who present with ACS at a younger age. Among patients with myocardial infarction, MetS is associated with worse in-hospital adverse outcomes, especially severe heart failure.[15] Patients with ACS and MetS should be targeted for aggressive lifestyle and risk factor modification.

Chronic kidney disease in ACS

Chronic kidney disease (CKD) is highly prevalent in patients with ACS and is associated with poor outcomes.[16] The observational SYCOMORE study found that one-third of patients presenting with ACS to a French university hospital had a creatinine clearance < 60 ml/min.[17] After adjusting for confounders, the study found that decreased renal function was independently associated with higher rates of in-hospital death and bleeding complications. Similarly, data from the SYMPHONY studies showed that for patients with ACS, whose creatinine clearance (CrCl) is ≤91 ml/min, each 10 ml/min increase in CrCl was associated with a 10% decrease in mortality.[18] At the same time, this study also found that patients with CKD and ACS were less often treated with aspirin, beta-blockers, unfractionated heparin, and statins.

Patients with CKD are at an increased risk for contrast-induced nephropathy (CIN) when undergoing coronary angiography. The iodinated contrast dyes used for imaging in the catheterization laboratory are nephrotoxic, and patients with CKD are at high risk for a deterioration of renal function following exposure. In most cases, CIN involves an asymptomatic rise in plasma creatinine concentration without permanent sequelae. In rare cases, however, CIN may progress to end-stage renal disease and need for hemodialysis. No specific treatment for CIN has proven beneficial; thus the primary focus is on prevention. The simplest method of prevention is avoidance of contrast media where possible. Patients with CKD should be carefully selected for angiography and should have limited exposure to contrast media during the procedure. Other preventative measures include avoidance of volume depletion and nonsteroidal anti-inflammatory drugs. Beyond this, several therapeutic measures have shown benefit in clinical trials for prevention of CIN. These are summarized in Table 5.3.

Table 5.3 Preventative measures for contrast-induced nephropathy

Measure	Dose/administration
N-acetylcysteine	600 mg PO bid on the day before and the day of angiography
Sodium bicarbonate infusion[a]	3 mg/kg/h of isotonic bicarbonate solution for one hour before procedure followed by 1 mg/kg/h for 6 hours after procedure
Isotonic saline infusion	1 mg/kg/h for at least 2 hours and preferably 6–12 hours before procedure, and continued for 6–12 hours after procedure

[a] The randomized REMEDIAL trial found bicarbonate infusion superior to isotonic saline. At many centers, sodium bicarbonate is preferred to isotonic saline for "pre-hydration" before angiography, particularly for CKD patients.

The most important impact of CKD on therapy of ACS is in the need to adjust medications for renal function. The glomerular filtration rate, using once of the two commonly used formulae (Table 5.4), should be estimated for every patient admitted with ACS. As compared with a simplified MDRD equation, the Cockcroft–Gault equation provides higher estimated GFR in younger patients and lower estimated GFR in patients older than 70 years. Table 5.5 lists the dosing adjustments for recommended therapies for ACS in patients with CKD.

Table 5.4 Estimation of glomerular filtration rate (GFR) with common methods

Cockroft–Gault formula

$$GFR \ (ml/min) \ = \frac{(140 - age) \times mass \ (in \ kilograms) \times [0.85 \ if \ female]}{72 \times serum \ creatinine \ (in \ mg/dl)}$$

MDRD formula

$$eGFR = 186 \times serum \ creatinine^{-1.154} \times age^{-0.203} \times [1.21 \ if \ Black] \\ \times [0.742 \ if \ female]$$

Table 5.5 Adjustment of common ACS medications for patients with CKD

Medication	Creatinine clearance		
	30–50 ml/min	**<30 ml/min**	**Dialysis**
Aspirin	None		
Clopidogrel	None		
Beta-blockers	Metoprolol is often preferred in CKD patients due to hepatic metabolism.		
Unfractionated heparin	None		
LMWH	None	Once daily dosing instead of bid	Not FDA approved for use in dialysis patients and may cause severe bleeding
Glycoprotein IIB/IIIA Inhibitors	Decrease dose based on CrCl and specific IIB/IIIA agent	Decrease dose based on CrCl and specific IIB/IIIA agent	Eptifibatide contraindicated in dialysis patients
Bivalarudin	None	Decrease infusion rate to 1 mg/kg/h	Decrease infusion rate to 0.25 mg/kg/h
Statins	None	None	Avoid highest dose

Young patients with ACS

ACS can occur in patients aged less than 60 years, often termed "premature" coronary disease. Younger patients with CAD are more likely to have conventional risk factors than older patients. Smoking is the single most important modifiable risk factor seen in young patients. Glucose abnormalities are common and may be subtle, but frank diabetes is less prevalent than in older patients.[19] Aggressive risk factor modification is recommended for any young patients with ACS. If marked lipid abnormalities are discovered, screening of first-degree relatives is reasonable.

ACS in the setting of cocaine use

Myocardial ischemia and infarction are well-documented complication of cocaine use, and cocaine intoxication as a precipitant should be considered in any young patient with ACS.[20] When ACS occurs in cocaine users, symptom onset is typically within 3 hours of exposure, but may occur up to 4 days later. The syndrome ranges from ischemic chest pain with or without biomarker elevation to ST elevation with complete arterial occlusion. The mechanism of cocaine-induced MI involves coronary vasospasm, increased myocardial oxygen demand secondary to tachycardia, and increased platelet adhesion.[21]

Treatment for ST-elevation MI in the setting of cocaine is the same as in patients without cocaine use. Aspirin, beta-blockers, heparin, IIB/IIIA inhibitors, and thrombolysis or PCI are indicated. For patients without ST elevation, management is often conservative, since as many as 40% of patients with cocaine-associated ACS have angiographically normal coronary arteries. The ACC/AHA has released guidelines for management of patients with chest pain after cocaine use (Table 5.6).[22] In contrast to noncocaine-

Table 5.6 ACC/AHA recommended therapies for cocaine-associated chest pain

Class I	Class II	Class III
• Benzodiazepines	• Calcium channel blockers	• Beta-blockers
• Aspirin	• Phentolamine	• Labetalol
• Nitroglycerin		

associated chest pain, benzodiazepines can be used (IB) and selective beta-blockers should be avoided (IIIC). In the setting of cocaine use, benzodiazepines relive chest pain and favorably effect hemodynamics, apparently through anxiolyitc properties and inhibition of the central stimulatory effects of cocaine. Beta-blockers may precipitate unopposed α-adrenergic effects in the setting of cocaine. This may lead to coronary vasoconstriction and elevated blood pressure. An overall treatment strategy is outlined in Figure 5.2.

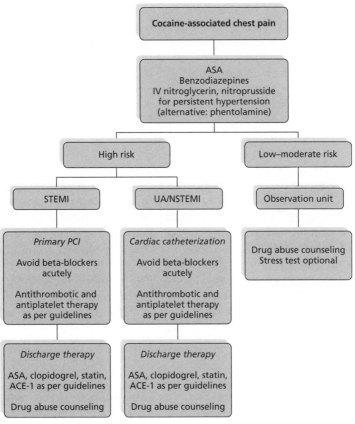

Figure 5.2 Diagnostic and therapeutic strategies in cocaine-associated chest pain (adapted, with permission, from McCord et al. Circulation 2008; 117: 1897–907[22]).

ACS in patients with normal coronary arteries or mild CAD

In clinical trials of non-ST-elevation ACS, 9–14% of patients have either normal vessels or no vessel with $\geq$50–60% stenosis on coronary angiography (so-called "mild" CAD, since at least 70% obstruction is necessary to limit blood flow). There are several possible mechanisms for these findings including rapid clot lysis, vasospasm, and coronary microvascular disease.

Patients with non-ST-elevation ACS with mild or no coronary artery disease have lower rates of adverse events than patients with critical lesions. For example, in a sub-study of the PURSUIT trial, the 30-day rate of death or myocardial infarction was significantly higher among patients with significant CAD (10%) compared to those with nonsignificant CAD (1.4%) or no CAD (0.9%).[23] In this trial, the strongest independent predictors of insignificant coronary disease were as follows:

- Female gender.
- Younger age (significant ↑ in likelihood of mild CAD per10-year ↓ in age).
- Absence of prior angina or diabetes.
- Absence of ST-segment depression or positive biomarkers.

Other data suggest that although short-term event rates are low, the long-term risk of adverse events in patients with no or mild CAD may still be high. A pooled analysis of non-ST-segment ACS from three TIMI trials (TIMI 11B, TIMI 16, and TIMI 22) found that 9.1% of patients had normal or nonobstructed coronary disease. The primary endpoint of death, MI, unstable angina requiring hospitalization, revascularization, or stroke occurred in 12% of this group at 1 year.[24]

Myocarditis

Myocarditis is a general term for inflammation of the myocardium. The term is usually invoked when inflammation of the myocardium occurs due to causes other than atherosclerosis and infarction. In developed countries, infection with Coxsackie B virus is the most common etiology.

Myocarditis is an important consideration in patients with ACS, since it can mimic an ischemic syndrome. Chest pain symptoms, ECG changes, biomarker elevation, and even wall motion abnormalities on echocardiogram can be identical to those of an ACS. Myocarditis should be suspected in a patient with a history of a recent viral syndrome (upper respiratory symptoms, fever, malaise), particularly if few risk factors for CAD are present.[25] If the pericardium is also inflamed (pericarditis), typical ECG changes of pericarditis, including diffuse ST elevation and PR depression, may occur. It is important to note, however, that myocarditis is a diagnosis of exclusion. Distinguishing the signs and symptoms apart from an ACS can be difficult. Ischemic heart disease should be the working diagnosis in any patient with signs and symptoms of ACS, and myocarditis should only be considered once CAD has been effectively ruled out as a cause. Cardiac MRI can be helpful in diagnosis and can show focal myocardial edema and late gadoliniuim enhancement in a noncoronary distribution. Coronary MRI can effectively rule out left main or three-vessel CAD as part of the same study.

Acute transient apical ballooning syndrome

Transient apical ballooning (also known as Takotsubo cardiomyopathy) is a syndrome characterized by apical left ventricular dysfunction that mimics myocardial infarction, often in the absence of significant coronary artery disease.[26] It is an important consideration in patients with acute chest pain, since the signs and symptoms are identical to those of an ACS.

The syndrome typically occurs in patients following a severe emotional stress. Symptoms usually include substernal chest pain, although some patients present with dyspnea or shock. The ECG will often show ST elevation in the anterior leads although other ECG abnormalities have been described. Cardiac biomarkers are frequently elevated. Imaging of the heart by echocardiography, left ventriuclography, or cardiac MRI show reduced LV function with akinesis or dyskinesis of the apical one-half to two-thirds of the heart.[27] Of particular importance, angiography in these patients may demonstrate normal coronary arteries or non-critical coronary disease. As with myocarditis, this is a diagnosis of exclusion, since distinguishing the disorder apart from an ACS with involvement of the mid- or distal LAD is often difficult. Most patients are taken for urgent catheterization for a presumed ST-elevation MI. They receive the diagnosis of apical ballooning syndrome only when the coronary arteries have no obstructive lesions and ventriculography shows the typical pattern. For patients who survive the acute episode, the disorder is usually self-limited. Left ventricular function typically recovers within 1–4 weeks.

Postoperative ACS

In the immediate postoperative period, patients who have undergone noncardiac surgery are at increased risk for myocardial infarction. Through changes in fluid balance, hemodynamic parameters, thrombogenicity, and adrenergic tone, surgical intervention predisposes to acute MI. For this reason, patients with risk factors for ACS should undergo a thorough evaluation prior to surgery with the aim of minimizing risk of cardiac complications. The pre-operative evaluation is a stepwise, guideline-driven process, which is well-outlined elsewhere.[28]

When acute MI occurs in the early postoperative period, attention is directed towards optimizing hemodynamics. Beta-blockers and nitrates are generally safe. Aspirin is generally acceptable, but the risk of bleeding with heparin and IIb/IIIa inhibitors in the first 48 hours following major surgery almost always outweighs the benefits of these medications. Percutaneous coronary revascularization is occasionally used, but stent implantation necessitates intensive and prolonged antiplatelet therapy, and is thus frequently unacceptable. Balloon angioplasty without stent implantation is a viable option in some of these cases. The input of the primary surgical team is essential in defining the bleeding risk associated with standard ACS therapies and prescribing the best course of action in a particular case.

ACS in a pregnant woman

Myocardial infarction (ST-elevation and non-ST-elevation) can occur in the peripartum period. The incidence is very low, although it may be slightly higher than for age-matched, nonpregnant women. A report from California found that from 1991 through 2000, there were 151 cases of pregnancy complicated by acute MI, resulting in an incidence of 2.8 per 100,000 deliveries.[29]

Most cases of peripartum MI occur in the third trimester or within 6 weeks postpartum. The anterior wall is commonly involved. The major risk factors appear to be older age, hypertension, and diabetes.

The mechanism of acute MI during pregnancy may be different that in nonpregnant patients. One study found that underlying atherosclerosis was present in less than half of cases.[30] The same study found that 21% of cases had normal coronary arteries, with a superimposed thrombus suggesting that hypercoaguability may play a role.

Spontaneous **coronary artery dissection** as a cause of acute MI appears to be more common during pregnancy. It most often occurs in the immediate peripartum period and is more frequent among mothers with hypertension. Initial ECG often demonstrates ST elevation, and management is the same as for other causes of ST-elevation MI. Because dissection of the arterial wall usually causes vessel occlusion, management typically involves percutaneous coronary intervention to restore flow to the myocardium.

The management of ACS during pregnancy is generally similar to that of nonpregnant patients with caveats for certain medications (Table 5.7). In most cases, a plan for urgent delivery of the fetus should be made in case of deterioration in maternal condition. Because of the hemodynamic stress associated with labor and delivery, some clinicians recommend delaying birth for 2–3 weeks after an MI if possible. Others recommend a cesarean section to minimize the workload for the mother. No randomized clinical trials have prospectively assessed timing or method of delivery after pregnancy-related MI.

In cases with minimal symptoms and only mild elevation of biomarkers, patients can be managed expectantly with

Table 5.7 ACS medications in pregnancy

Medication	Pregnancy class	Comment
Aspirin	C	A low dose of aspirin (75–162 mg/day) appears to be safe
Heparin	C	Does not cross placenta; safe for fetus, but maternal bleeding may occur
Nitrates	C	Generally safe, although maternal hypotension must be avoided
Beta-blockers	C	Often used, although occasional cases of fetal growth restriction, hypoglycemia, respiratory depression, and bradycardia have been reported
ACE inhibitors	D	Contraindicated
Statins	X	Contraindicated
Thrombolytics	C	Relatively contraindicated due to high rates of maternal bleeding; some women have been safely treated
Clopidogrel	B	Limited experience in pregnancy
IIB/IIIA inhibitors	B	Limited experience in pregnancy
Direct thrombin inhibitors	B	Limited experience in pregnancy

aspirin, beta-blockers, and heparin. When severe symptoms, hemodynamic compromise, or ST elevations are present, urgent revascularization with PCI is usually indicated. There are no controlled studies examining thrombolysis during pregnancy, and pregnancy is considered a relative contraindication to thrombolysis in the 2004 American College of Cardiology Guidelines.

Hyperthyroidism and ACS

Hyperthyroidism leads to increased heart rate, myocardial contractility, and myocardial oxygen demand, which can precipitate angina in patients with coronary stenoses. Elevated thyroid hormone levels can also directly cause coronary vasospasm. Hyperthyroidism should be considered in patients with known stable angina who develop accelerating symptoms. Moreover, in patients with new-onset angina or ACS, hyperthyroidism may be a precipitating factor.

ACS in patients exposed to radiation

Radiation therapy directed at the chest is routinely used to treat malignancies such as breast cancer and lymphoma. When coronary stenoses develop following radiation, they typically involve the proximal portions of the LAD and RCA vessels, since these receive the highest radiation exposure. Various forms of ACS ranging from angina to sudden cardiac death have been reported.

Trauma and ACS

Rarely, myocardial infarction may complicate blunt chest wall trauma. Case reports have demonstrated causes such as coronary artery dissection and thrombosis. The LAD appears to be most frequently involved, although any coronary artery may be affected. Few data are available to guide treatment, due to the rare nature of the disorder. Coronary angiography with stenting may be appropriate. Thrombolysis has been successfully used, but it may lead to severe bleeding depending on the nature of the trauma.

ACS because of coronary occlusion in trauma may be difficult to differentiate from **cardiac contusion**, which can also present with chest pain, ECG abnormalities, and cardiac biomarker release. However, unlike ACS, cardiac contusion is caused by direct trauma to the myocardium, often from blunt contact with the chest wall. This condition is generally treated with supportive care, and patients are monitored for development of arrhythmia in the early post-trauma period.

References

1. Haffner SM, Lehto S, Ronnemaa T, Pyorala K, Laakso M. Mortality from coronary heart disease in subjects with type 2 diabetes and in nondiabetic subjects with and without prior myocardial infarction. *N Engl J Med* 1998; 339: 229–34.
2. Juutilainen A, Lehto S, Ronnemaa T, Pyorala K, Laakso M. Type 2 diabetes as a "coronary heart disease equivalent": an 18-year

prospective population-based study in Finnish subjects. *Diabetes Care* 2005; 28: 2901–7.

3. Mak KH, Topol EJ. Emerging concepts in the management of acute myocardial infarction in patients with diabetes mellitus. *J Am Coll Cardiol* 2000; 35: 563–8.

4. Granger CB, Califf RM, Young S, *et al*. Outcome of patients with diabetes mellitus and acute myocardial infarction treated with thrombolytic agents. The Thrombolysis and Angioplasty in Myocardial Infarction (TAMI) Study Group. *J Am Coll Cardiol* 1993; 21: 920–5.

5. Mak KH, Moliterno DJ, Granger CB, *et al*. Influence of diabetes mellitus on clinical outcome in the thrombolytic era of acute myocardial infarction. GUSTO-I Investigators. Global Utilization of Streptokinase and Tissue Plasminogen Activator for Occluded Coronary Arteries. *J Am Coll Cardiol* 1997; 30: 171–9.

6. Malmberg K, Ryden L, Efendic S, *et al*. Randomized trial of insulin-glucose infusion followed by subcutaneous insulin treatment in diabetic patients with acute myocardial infarction (DIGAMI study): effects on mortality at 1 year. *J Am Coll Cardiol* 1995; 26: 57–65.

7. Malmberg K, Ryden L, Wedel H, *et al*. Intense metabolic control by means of insulin in patients with diabetes mellitus and acute myocardial infarction (DIGAMI 2): effects on mortality and morbidity. *Eur Heart J* 2005; 26: 650–61.

8. Mehta SR, Yusuf S, Diaz R, *et al*. Effect of glucose-insulin-potassium infusion on mortality in patients with acute ST-segment elevation myocardial infarction: the CREATE-ECLA randomized controlled trial. *Jama* 2005; 293: 437–46.

9. Antman EM, Anbe DT, Armstrong PW, *et al*. ACC/AHA guidelines for the management of patients with ST-elevation myocardial infarction—executive summary. A report of the American College of Cardiology/American Heart Association Task Force on Practice Guidelines (Writing Committee to revise the 1999 guidelines for the management of patients with acute myocardial infarction). *J Am Coll Cardiol* 2004; 44: 671–719.

10. Influence of diabetes on 5-year mortality and morbidity in a randomized trial comparing CABG and PTCA in patients with multivessel disease: the Bypass Angioplasty Revascularization Investigation (BARI). *Circulation* 1997; 96: 1761–9.

11. Serruys PW, Unger F, Sousa JE, *et al*. Comparison of coronary-artery bypass surgery and stenting for the treatment of multivessel disease. *N Engl J Med* 2001; 344: 1117–24.

12. Kapur A. Coronary artery revascularization in diabetics: The CARDia trial. *Presented at the European Society of Cardiology, Munich, Germany, August/September 2008.*

13. Serruys PW. The synergy between percutaneous coronary intervention with TAXUS and cardiac surgery: The SYNTAX study. *Presented at the European Society of Cardiology Congress, Munich, Germany, August/September 2008.*

14. Executive Summary of the Third Report of the National Cholesterol Education Program (NCEP) Expert Panel on Detection, Evaluation, and Treatment of High Blood Cholesterol In Adults (Adult Treatment Panel III). *Jama* 2001; 285: 2486–97.

15. Zeller M, Steg PG, Ravisy J, *et al*. Prevalence and impact of metabolic syndrome on hospital outcomes in acute myocardial infarction. *Arch Intern Med* 2005; 165: 1192–8.

16. Freeman RV, Mehta RH, Al Badr W, Cooper JV, Kline-Rogers E, Eagle KA. Influence of concurrent renal dysfunction on outcomes of patients with acute coronary syndromes and implications of the use of glycoprotein IIb/IIIa inhibitors. *J Am Coll Cardiol* 2003; 41: 718–24.

17. Dumaine R, Collet JP, Tanguy ML, *et al*. Prognostic significance of renal insufficiency in patients presenting with acute coronary syndrome (the Prospective Multicenter SYCOMORE study). *Am J Cardiol* 2004; 94: 1543–7.

18. Reddan DN, Szczech L, Bhapkar MV, *et al*. Renal function, concomitant medication use and outcomes following acute coronary syndromes. *Nephrol Dial Transplant* 2005; 20: 2105–12.

19. Chouhan L, Hajar HA, Pomposiello JC. Comparison of thrombolytic therapy for acute myocardial infarction in patients aged <35 and >55 years. *Am J Cardiol* 1993; 71: 157–9.

20. Hollander JE, Hoffman RS, Gennis P, *et al*. Prospective multicenter evaluation of cocaine-associated chest pain. Cocaine Associated Chest Pain (COCHPA) Study Group. *Acad Emerg Med* 1994; 1: 330–9.

21. Gradman AH. Cardiac effects of cocaine: a review. *Yale J Biol Med* 1988; 61: 137–47.

22. McCord J, Jneid H, Hollander JE, *et al*. Management of cocaine-associated chest pain and myocardial infarction: a scientific statement from the American Heart Association Acute Cardiac Care Committee of the Council on Clinical Cardiology. *Circulation* 2008; 117: 1897–907.

23. Roe MT, Harrington RA, Prosper DM, *et al*. Clinical and therapeutic profile of patients presenting with acute coronary syndromes who do not have significant coronary artery disease. The Platelet Glycoprotein IIb/IIIa in Unstable Angina: Receptor Suppression Using Integrilin Therapy (PURSUIT) Trial Investigators. *Circulation* 2000; 102: 1101–6.

24. Bugiardini R, Manfrini O, De Ferrari GM. Unanswered questions for management of acute coronary syndrome: risk stratification of

patients with minimal disease or normal findings on coronary angiography. *Arch Intern Med* 2006; 166: 1391–5.

25. Dennert R, Crijns HJ, Heymans S. Acute viral myocarditis. *Eur Heart J* 2008; 29: 2073–82.

26. Bybee KA, Kara T, Prasad A, *et al.* Systematic review: transient left ventricular apical ballooning: a syndrome that mimics ST-segment elevation myocardial infarction. *Ann Intern Med* 2004; 141: 858–65.

27. Koeth O, Mark B, Kilkowski A, *et al.* Clinical, angiographic and cardiovascular magnetic resonance findings in consecutive patients with Takotsubo cardiomyopathy. *Clin Res Cardiol* 2008; 97: 623–7.

28. Fleisher LA, Beckman JA, Brown KA, *et al.* ACC/AHA 2007 guidelines on perioperative cardiovascular evaluation and care for noncardiac surgery: a report of the American College of Cardiology/American Heart Association Task Force on Practice Guidelines (Writing Committee to Revise the 2002 Guidelines on Perioperative Cardiovascular Evaluation for Noncardiac Surgery) developed in collaboration with the American Society of Echocardiography, American Society of Nuclear Cardiology, Heart Rhythm Society, Society of Cardiovascular Anesthesiologists, Society for Cardiovascular Angiography and Interventions, Society for Vascular Medicine and Biology, and Society for Vascular Surgery. *J Am Coll Cardiol* 2007; 50: e159–e241.

29. Ladner HE, Danielsen B, Gilbert WM. Acute myocardial infarction in pregnancy and the puerperium: a population-based study. *Obstet Gynecol* 2005; 105: 480–4.

30. Roth A, Elkayam U. Acute myocardial infarction associated with pregnancy. *Ann Intern Med* 1996; 125: 751–62.

CHAPTER 6

Complications of acute coronary syndrome

Jan M. Pattanayak and Eli V. Gelfand

Introduction

The in-hospital mortality in patients with acute myocardial infarction has steadily declined over the last several decades to <10%.[1] This remarkable achievement is due to the development of rapid pharmacologic and mechanical reperfusion and adjunctive pharmacotherapy, as well as to the development of rapid cardiac referral networks and coronary care units. Despite these advances, myocardial infarction remains a life-threatening illness, and a busy clinician must be acutely aware of a number of important complications. Likewise, newer therapies for ACS, such as percutaneous coronary interventions, have become increasingly complex and inherently carry their own risk of complications.

Thus, while general management principles of acute coronary syndromes are discussed in Chapters 3 and 4, this chapter is dedicated specifically to the diagnosis and management of complications of both ACS itself and therapies for ACS.

Pump failure

General principle
Cardiogenic shock due to pump failure remains the most common cause of in-hospital demise in patients with acute

Management of Acute Coronary Syndromes   Eli V. Gelfand and Christopher P. Cannon
© 2009 John Wiley & Sons, Ltd

coronary syndrome. Data from the GUSTO-IIb trial suggests that cardiogenic shock complicates approximately 4% of acute STEMI and 2.5% of NSTEMI cases.[2] Overall, about 2% of ACS patients are in shock upon hospital presentation. In addition, despite primary reperfusion and adjunctive medical therapy, cardiogenic shock develops in some patients in the hospital. Latest registry data suggest that as ACS therapies advanced in the last 10 years, the rate of in-hospital cardiogenic shock fell by approximately 75% (from 10.6% to 2.7%).[3] The etiology of shock is usually progressive infarction of the LV, although RV infarct or mechanical myocardial complications may be a separate primary cause, and are discussed henceforth. Although the mortality in patients with cardiogenic shock from LV infarction has fallen from 90% prior to introduction of reperfusion therapy, it continues to be over 50% in the era of widespread thrombolytic therapy and PCI.[4]

Clinical presentation

The clinical hallmark of cardiogenic shock is diminished end-organ perfusion, which manifests as cool, clammy extremities, oliguria with urine output <20 ml/h, and diminished mental alertness. The filling pressures are usually elevated with pulmonary capillary wedge pressure exceeding 25 mmHg, a cardiac index of <2 l/min/m^2, and systolic arterial pressure <90 mmHg (mean, <60 mmHg). As the LV stroke volume falls due to worsening contractile function, compensatory tachycardia develops, diastolic period shortens, and LV filling is further impaired. The Killip classification of CHF (Table 6.1) reflects the outward manifestations of acute MI hemodynamics. This 40-year-old classification remains useful in clinical management of patients with complicated MI, largely because of its simplicity.

Most patients will not present with pump failure on hospital admission, but will develop it in the hospital. Progressive pump failure then puts into motion a series of pathophysiologic events, which lead to worsening coronary perfusion and more pump failure (Figure 6.1).

Table 6.1 The Killip classification of patients with acute MI (adapted from Killip et al.[5])

Classification	Examination findings	Typical findings on right heart catheterization
I	No clinical signs of heart failure	Normal hemodynamics
II	Basilar rales, S_3 gallop	Elevated PCWP, normal CO/CI
III	• Rales over >50% of lung fields • Pulmonary edema	• Further elevated PCWP • Normal or slightly reduced CO/CI
IV	Cardiogenic shock: • Rales • Cool, clammy extremities • Relative hypotension • Decreased urine output • Altered mental status	• Elevated PCWP • Reduced CO/CI

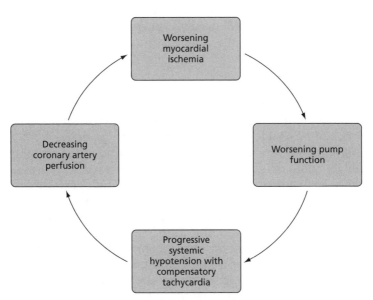

Figure 6.1 The "vicious cycle" of cardiogenic shock.

Prognosis

The prognosis in cardiogenic shock has improved recently, mostly because of more rapid and effective reperfusion. The pivotal SHOCK trial enrolled 302 patients presenting with cardiogenic shock within 36 hours of acute MI and randomized them to emergency revascularization (within 6 hours) or initial medical stabilization with delayed (after 54 hours) revascularization.[3] Although the primary endpoint of all-cause mortality at 30 days did not reach clinical significance (53% survived with emergency revascularization vs. 44% with delayed), the secondary endpoint of mortality at 6 months was significantly better with the emergency versus delayed reperfusion (survival of 50% vs. 37%, respectively). In a subgroup analysis, patients <75 years old benefited from early revascularization both at 30 days and 6 months. In this cohort, 20 lives were saved at 6 months for every 100 subjects treated emergently. In a series of 200 patients admitted with acute MI complicated by cardiogenic shock, in-hospital mortality was 53%, and the predictors of mortality were larger size of the infarct (as determined by peak CK levels) and lack of TIMI grade 3 flow in the infarct-related artery.[6]

Treatment

Circulatory support in cardiogenic shock

Management of most patients with progressive cardiogenic shock after AMI is often made easier with guidance from a pulmonary artery catheter (PAC). In addition to providing reliable data on intracardiac filling pressures, vascular resistance and cardiac output, a PAC allows for quick assessment of the response to treatment of shock and rapid detection of mechanical complications of ACS. Specific guidelines for invasive hemodynamic monitoring in acute MI are available in the ACC/AHA guidelines, and recommend PA catheter for progressive hypotension when unresponsive to fluid administration or when fluid administration is contraindicated (i.e., pulmonary edema)

First, the volume status of the patient must be optimized. Previously healthy patients with an acute MI are unlikely to be chronically volume-overloaded. In fact, the presenting symptom of dyspnea in these diuretic-naïve patients is often presumptively managed with large doses of loop diuretics during initial medical contact, and relative hypovolemia is not an uncommon phenomenon in the ensuing several hours. When replacing intravascular volume in these patients, a pulmonary capillary wedge pressure (PCWP) of 18–20 mmHg is a reasonable goal, since under these conditions the cardiac output should be maximized. Further administration of fluids in response to arterial hypotension is only likely to lead to pulmonary edema, and other explanation for hypotension, such as diminishing cardiac output, mechanical complication of MI, or concomitant distributive shock should be sought. If cardiac output remains low after optimization of filling pressures and afterload, inotropic agents such as dobutamine, milrinone, or dopamine are considered, with the choice of specific agent guided by patient's hemodynamic profile and the drug's known physiologic effects (Table 6.2).

Most inotropic agents worsen ischemia and are intrinsically arrhythmogenic. Hence, if cardiogenic shock persists despite complete revascularization and best medical care, strong consideration should be given to placement of a mechanical assist device. These range from the percutaneously implanted and easily removable intraaortic balloon pump (IABP) to surgically placed ventricular assist devices (VAD), and even complete bypass of the heart and lungs in the form of an extracorporeal membrane oxygenation (ECMO) system. The last two options are rarely used, are reserved for extreme cases, and usually involve concomitant evaluation for urgent cardiac transplantation. These devices are summarized in Table 6.3, and a primer on IABP can be found in the Appendix.

Supportive therapy in cardiogenic shock

Hypoxemia and acidosis are frequent comordibities in cardiogenic shock, and should be diagnosed and treated aggressively. Frequent arterial blood gas monitoring is made easier and more comfortable for the patient by placing an indwelling radial arterial catheter, which is also used for continuous blood pressure monitoring. Hypoxemia is usually a consequence of pulmonary edema and negatively

Table 6.2 Major physiologic effects of hemodynamically active agents commonly used in treating complicated acute MI

Agent	Dose	Hemodynamic effects	Side effects
Dobutamine	2–10 mcg/kg/min	• Increased CO • Increased contractility • Decreases SVR and PVR	• Tachycardia • Hypotension if SVR falls more than CO rises • Tachyarrhythmias
Dopamine	5–10 mcg/kg/min	• Increased CO • Increased contractility • Vasoconstriction at higher doses • Possible increased renal perfusion	• Tachycardia • Arrhythimias
Milrinone	0.25–0.750 mcg/kg/min after a slow bolus of 50 mcg/kg	• Increased CO • Decreased SVR and PVR	• Tachyarrhythmia • 2.5 hour half-life
Norepinephirine	5–30 mcg/min	• Increased CO • Increased SVR	• Increased myocardial oxygen demand • Coronary vasoconstriction
Nitroglycerin	0–100 mcg/min	• Arterial and venous vasodilation with decreased SVR and PVR	• Hypotension • Severe hypotension if RV involvement • Headache
Nitroprusside	0.5–10.0 mcg/kg/min; but high doses only to be used for very short durations	• Vasodilation with decreased SVR	• Cyanide toxicity with long-term administration • Worsening V/Q mismatch via pulmonary vasodilation

Table 6.3 Mechanical support devices for acute MI

Device	Benefits	Limitations
IABP	• Increased coronary artery perfusion with a drop in SVR and an increase in CO causing increased BP • Can be inserted quickly in all interventional catheterization laboratories • Useful for stabilizing patients prior to performing the intervention	• Vascular complications • Infection risk • Bleeding risk, as requires heparin
Standard ventricular assist device (VAD)	• Long-term unloading of the ventricle in patients with progressive refractory shock • Can be used as a destination or as a bridge to transplant	• Specialized centers only • Cost • Infection • Clot and stroke risk
Percutaneous VAD	• Percutaneously inserted VAD with inflow via LA catheter, with outflow into the femoral artery • Allows a greater degree of support than IABP	• Not yet widely available • Requires trans-septal puncture to place the LA catheter
Extra-corporeal membranous oxygenation (ECMO)	• Total unloading of the ventricle and lungs	• Can only be performed in experienced centers with cardiac surgery • Vascular complications • Risk of stroke

impacts oxygen delivery to the recovering myocardium. Treatment of hypoxemia may necessitate mechanical ventilation. Tachypnea *without* frank hypoxemia in the setting of cardiogenic shock often reflects an appropriate respiratory compensation of lactic acidosis, and is best approached by correcting the underlying hypoperfusion.

Untreated acidosis, particularly with arterial blood pH < 7.30, reduces myocardial contractility, decreases responsiveness to inotropic therapy, and promotes the vicious cycle of cardiogenic shock. Sodium bicarbonate will correct acidosis at the expense of hypernatremia and hypervolemia, and therefore is not used unless acidosis is profound (pH < 7.10). Instead, gradual correction of acidosis is achieved by improving organ perfusion with inotropic agents, and supporting respiratory compensation. Tracheal intubation with hyperventilation may be necessary if respiratory fatigue develops.

Right ventricular infarction

Introduction
The majority of the right ventricular free wall is supplied by the marginal branch of the right coronary artery. Portions of the inferior and posterior free wall are served by the poster-ior descending branch of the RCA. Thus, right ventricular myocardial infarction (RVMI) is typically a consequence of a proximal RCA occlusion. Furthermore, the anterior portion of the free wall may have additional blood supply from the moderator branch of the left anterior descending artery.

Right ventricular infarction should be suspected in any patient with an acute MI involving the inferior and/or pos-terior walls. In general, because of its smaller muscle mass and its continuous (diastolic *and* systolic) coronary perfu-sion, the RV is less susceptible to ischemia. Overall, *combined* RV and LV infarction is the rule, with *isolated* RV infarction found in <5% of cases.

Clinical presentation
Patients with RVMI are often acutely ill during their initial hospital course, including in the immediate hours after PCI/fibrinolysis, due to the hemodynamic consequences stem-ming from the loss of RV contractile function. However, once the coronary occlusion is reperfused, RV systolic func-tion typically improves, even if regional akinesis was present on the early imaging study. This is in contrast to LV infarction, where improvement in severe regional LV dysfunction is less predictable, and more dependent on rapid reperfusion.

Typical symptoms of concomitant acute LV myocardial infarction usually predominate, with chest pain, dyspnea, and tachycardia. In cases of isolated RV infarction, there is acute RV diastolic dysfunction, with reduced ventricular fill-ing, increased right-sided pressures and RV dilation, and a subsequent decrease in RV output, leading to the reduction in LV filling and, thus, to a decrease in LV output. Because the left-sided filling pressure is initially normal, such patients are observed to have jugular venous distention with lack of JVP collapse on inspiration (Kussmaul's sign) and hypotension with clear lung fields. This presentation may be initially confused with pulmonary embolism or cardiac tamponade. However, initial testing, including EKG and echo, easily distinguishes between these entities. Patients with RV infarct often have prominent vagal symptoms with nausea/vomiting, and abdominal pain. These may occur with or without traditional chest pain. Sinus bradycardia or junctional rhythm and atrioventricular (AV) conduction abnormalities, including AV dissociation, are frequently seen.

Diagnosis

The first clues to an RV infarct on **electrocardiography** are signs of concomitant inferior LV STEMI, as evidenced by ST-segment elevations in the inferior leads (II, III, avF) (for more on ECG in the diagnosis of STEMI, see Chapter 2). Frequently, ST-segment elevation is also seen in lead V_1, which is placed directly over the RV in patients with normal anatomy (Figure 6.2).[7] Recognition of this pattern should prompt the performance of right-sided leads. ST-segment elevations in right-sided lead V_4 (V_4R) of ≥ 1 mm are found in almost 90% of patients with an RV infarct (Figure 6.3).[8] **Echocardiography** demonstrates regional RV hypokinesis and is useful in assessing the extent of the associated LV infarction. Invasive hemodynamic evaluation with **right heart catheterization** is often performed following primary angioplasty and can confirm the diagnosis of RV infarction. A frequently observed hemodynamic sign is an increase in RA pressure out of proportion to pulmonary capillary wedge pressure, so that the RA/PCWP ratio is ≥ 0.8 (normal, <0.6). Other hemodynamic findings include elevated RVEDP with a "dip and plateau" waveform (Figure 6.4) and a narrowed PA pulse pressure. Because of the reduced LV filling, cardiac output may be diminished, with a compensatory rise in systemic vascular resistance.

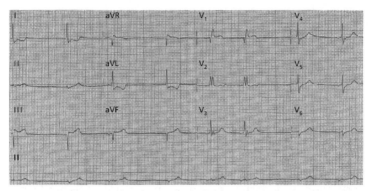

Figure 6.2 A 12-lead ECG in a patient with acute inferior MI, complicated by RVMI and shock. There is intermittent slow junctional rhythm and ST elevation in lead V₁ is seen.

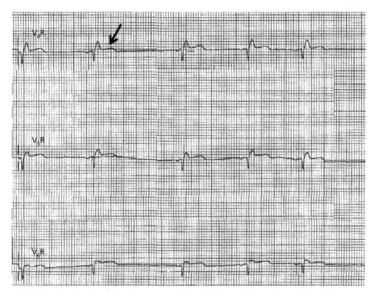

Figure 6.3 A 12-lead ECG in a patient with acute RVMI, showing ST-segment elevation in lead V₄R.

Management

Patients with RV infarct physiology are dependent on the systemic preload to maintain RV filling and thus to deliver oxygenated blood to the left heart. As such, interventions that decrease central venous pressure may result in a marked

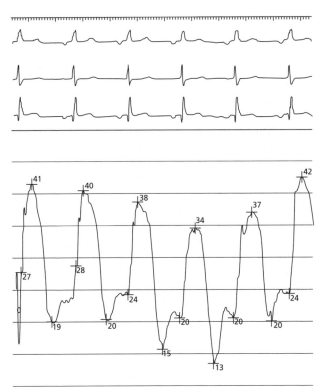

Figure 6.4 A right ventricular pressure tracing, showing elevated RVEDP with a characteristic "dip and plateau" waveform.

reduction in cardiac output and may precipitate systemic hypotension. Nitrates and morphine should be used with caution. A rapid drop in blood pressure in response to a nitrate in patients with inferior STEMI should immediately alert the clinician to the possibility of RV involvement. Reperfusion strategy in patients with isolated RV infarction does not differ from general treatment strategy of STEMI—time to reperfusion is of the essence. With regard to hemodynamic management, patients with isolated RV infarction and hypotension may initially be managed with a small bolus infusion of normal saline to achieve a CVP of around 12 mmHg. In the absence of objective evidence of ongoing low RV filling pressures (collapsed jugular veins on physical examination, low CVP on invasive monitoring), administration of further fluids should be avoided, as further RV dilation contributes to ongoing ischemia. If hypotension persists despite adequate hydration, a inotropic agent such as dobutamine at a dose of 5–10 mcg/kg/min may be considered.[9]

Atrioventricular dyssynchrony in patients with RVMI is poorly tolerated, and in patients with high-grade AV block, the threshold for temporary sequential transvenous pacing should be low. Most of these patients will recover AV conduction within 24–48 hours. In patients with atrial fibrillation, sinus rhythm should be restored promptly with synchronized cardioversion.

Prognosis
In general, the presence of RV infarction confers a markedly higher risk of in-hospital death in patients with inferior LVMI. A meta-analysis of six studies involving 1,198 patients found that compared with subjects with LVMI only, those with an additional RVMI had a three-fold increase in each of the following events: ventricular tachyarrhythmia, AV block, shock, and death.[10]

Mechanical complications of ACS

Introduction
The three most frequent mechanical complications of acute MI are LV free wall rupture, ventricular septal rupture (VSR), and acute mitral regurgitation (MR) from papillary muscle rupture. The underlying cause of all three mechanical complications is essentially the same—transmural necrosis of an area of infarcted myocardium, with the creation of mechanical discontinuity in the left ventricle. Classically, these present 2–5 days into the course of the infarction, and present as sudden, unexpected hemodynamic deterioration. The incidence of mechanical complications has decreased with the advent of early reperfusion, but they remain a significant short-term cause of death in acute MI.

Left ventricular free wall rupture
Left ventricular free wall rupture occurs in 1–2% of patients with acute MI. The risk increases with age, female gender,

hypertension, and first presentation of MI. The first clinical presentation of CAD is likely a marker for lack of collateral formation, which subjects the area supplied by the infarct-related artery to a higher risk of transmural necrosis. The clinical presentation of free wall rupture follows one of two courses. Sudden hemodynamic collapse and electromechanical dissociation from acute hemopericardium is the typical presentation. Mortality is exceedingly high, and the only treatment is emergency surgery. A subset of patients will exhibit a more subacute presentation, with impending rupture suggested by episodes of chest pain (often with features suggesting pericarditis), nausea, vomiting, and diaphoresis. Rapid diagnosis with echocardiography, followed by emergency surgery, is lifesaving. Infrequently, such subacute presentation results in formation of thrombotic "seal" on the epicardial surface, which organizes into an **LV pseudoaneurysm** (see below).

Ventricular septal rupture
Ventricular septal rupture (VSR) complicates 2–4% of acute STEMI. In the setting of inferior MI, the resulting defect is often localized to the basal septum and is typically large. With anterior MI, the defect is frequently more apical and smaller. The risks of developing VSR are similar to those of free wall rupture, and may be particularly high in patients receiving fibrinolytics late after the onset of symptoms. The time course of VSR follows a bimodal distribution, with an increase in the first 24 hours in those receiving fibrinolysis, and a second peak 3–5 days after presentation. The clinical presentation of VSR depends greatly on the size of the defect, the pressure gradient between LV and RV, and the underlying ventricular function. Small defects may present with exacerbation of chest pain several days after reperfusion, but without overt heart failure. Large defects result in acute pulmonary hypertension with right heart failure from massive left-to-right shunting. The presence of a new harsh systolic murmur, accompanied by a thrill and an RV heave, should alert the clinician that a VSR may be present. Doppler echocardiography is able to confirm the vast majority of VSR and has an additional advantage of quantifying the size of the defect, evaluating pulmonary arterial pressures and

biventricular systolic function. If a PA catheter is in place, samples of blood from the right atrium and the right ventricle (or the pulmonary artery) can be obtained quickly, and will demonstrate a "step up" in oxygen saturation between the RA and PA. Definitive therapy of VSR in most cases is surgical closure. The tissue surrounding the postinfarct ventricular septal defect is necrotic, making surgical closure of a postinfarct ventricular septal defect a technically challenging procedure. However, unlike in free wall rupture, patients with VSR can often be initially managed medically, allowing for some degree of healing and remodeling, making the corrective surgery more reliable. Percutaneous closure of VSR is an emerging alternative to surgery, but outcomes are also better if the procedure can be safely delayed.

Acute mitral regurgitation

Acute mitral regurgitation in the setting of MI is almost always associated with rupture of a papillary muscle. This complication must be differentiated from **ischemic papillary muscle dysfunction**, which has a similar etiology, but does not involve an actual disarticulation of the papillary muscle head from the subtending LV wall. The anterolateral papillary muscle has dual blood supply from the left anterior descending and the left circumflex arteries, and is therefore less prone to ischemia than the posteromedial papillary muscle, which is typically supplied by a single dominant artery (right coronary or left circumflex). Consequently, papillary muscle rupture is seen more commonly as a complication of inferior infarction. The mitral valve is a complex three-dimensional structure, and a profound change in its mechanics, such as seen even in a partial papillary muscle tear, almost uniformly results in a flail mitral leaflet and severe MR. Clinically, the disorder is that of combined acute pulmonary venous hypertension resulting in pulmonary edema, and a sharp decrease in forward cardiac output, manifesting as cardiogenic shock. On examination, a new holosystolic murmur radiating to the back and axilla is appreciated, along with signs of acute pulmonary edema. Again, an echocardiogram with Doppler investigation can easily differentiate papillary muscle rupture with severe MR and a flail segment from VSD and from milder forms of ischemic MR. Management of acute MR consists of afterload reduction with pharmacologic (nitroprusside, nitroglycerin) and/or mechanical (IABP) means, followed by surgery. Inotropes (milrinone, dobutamine) may be temporarily given to patients in shock, while surgery is being arranged.

One algorithm for diagnosis and therapy of suspected mechanical complication of an acute MI is given below (Figure 6.5).

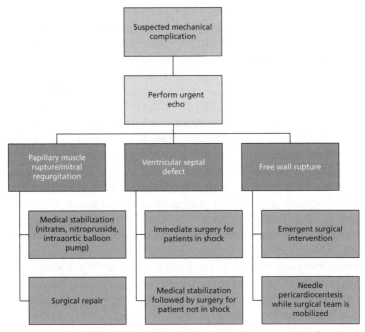

Figure 6.5 Suspected mechanical complications of myocardial infarction.

Left ventricular aneurysm

The natural history of acute MI with regional left ventricular systolic dysfunction involves expansion of the area of infarcted myocardium secondary to LV wall thinning and stretching. Eventually, the thin and noncontractile area of myocardium "bulges out" and may be frankly dyskinetic, moving *outward* in systole, thus forming a **left ventricular aneurysm**. The diagnosis of LV aneurysm is suggested on

ECG by the persistence of ST-segment elevations days to weeks following an acute MI, but confirmation with echocardiography or cardiac MRI is necessary. Complications of a ventricular aneurysm involve **thrombosis** with systemic embolization (SE), worsening of **heart failure**, and **ventricular tachyarrhythmias.**[11]

Left ventricular intracavitary thrombosis is usually seen with large anterior myocardial infarctions, stemming from LAD occlusion. The risk is highest in the first 48 hours, and the vast majority of thrombi will form within the first 10–14 days. An early trial compared high-dose with low-dose subcutaneous unfractionated heparin after acute anterior STEMI, and found a significant reduction in the occurrence of LV thrombus with high-dose heparin (11% vs. 32%, $p < 0.05$), without a difference in hemorrhagic complications.[12] An empiric strategy of systemic anticoagulation with warfarin is theoretically attractive, but it is associated with significant bleeding risks, especially when administered concomitantly with dual antiplatelet therapy. Randomized trials of anticoagulation to prevent SE following acute MI are lacking, but a meta-analysis of several observational studies confirms a high incidence of SE in patients with anterior MI, and generally supports warfarin anticoagulation for several months after the index event.[13] Therefore, the current ACC/AHA guidelines recommend at least 3 months of warfarin for patients with LV thrombus noted on imaging study, and indefinitely in patients without an increased level of bleeding. Furthermore, the guidelines give a recommendation for warfarin in post-STEMI patients with extensive regional wall-motion abnormalities and LV dysfunction.[14,15] A more detailed discussion of clinical trials of anticoagulation following ACS is included in Chapter 7. At our institution, the early anticoagulation strategy involves risk stratification with echocardiography shortly following acute MI. Patients in whom involvement of a large portion of the anterior wall/apex is suspected on the basis of timing of presentation and angiographic outcomes are typically continued on an IV heparin infusion pending echocardiography, so that in these patients, there is no gap in anticoagulation.

Surgical resection of an aneurysm (aneurysmectomy) can be performed at the time of CABG. The current guidelines recommend that aneurysmectomy be considered in patients with an LV aneurysm, who have intractable heart failure or ventricular tachyarrhythmias. Concurrent revascularization should be performed when feasible. For patients with incessant, poorly tolerated ventricular tachycardia (VT), additional endocardial mapping and ablation of the arrhythmic substrate can be combined with aneurysmectomy and bypass grafting.[16]

Left ventricular pseudoaneurysm

Left ventricular pseudoaneurysm (LVPsA; false LV aneurysm) is rupture of the free LV wall, contained by adjacent epicardial clot, scar, and adherent pericardial tissue. The hallmark symptoms of LVPsA are chest pain and dyspnea, although up to 25% of patients are asymptomatic.[17] Physical examination may reveal heart failure, a machinery-like murmur secondary to flow in and out of the PsA, and—occasionally—a pericardial rub. Because the rupture is by definition contained, frank tamponade is uncommon, although loculated hemopericardium may infrequently exert significant external pressure on the left ventricle. A diagnosis can be made on echocardiography, but—if feasible—a cardiac MRI provides the best anatomic definition of the defect. In a single comprehensive examination, cardiac MRI can distinguish between a true LV aneurysm and LVPsA, quantify LV global and regional systolic function, assess myocardial viability, and define coronary anatomy.

Mortality in LVPsA without treatment is substantial, and patients should be referred for surgical repair. As in surgical therapy of true LV aneurysms, coronary revascularization, when feasible, should be performed along with the primary repair.

Pericardial complications

Early postinfarction pericarditis may occur within days of a transmural MI, especially if the time to reperfusion was prolonged. The pathophysiology has not been well-elucidated, but presumably relates to local inflammation which accompanies healing of the acute infarct. The clinical presentation is that of chest pain, and is differentiated from postinfarct angina or recurrent MI on the basis of ECG changes of diffuse concave ST elevations, seen in a noncoronary distribution. Elevation of the PR segments in lead aVR, and PR segment depressions in the other leads are frequently seen. A triphasic pericardial friction rub may be auscultated.

Early pericarditis is distinguished from **late postinfarction pericarditis**, alternatively termed **Dressler's syndrome** or post-cardiac injury syndrome, which typically presents *weeks* after the index event. This syndrome can also occur after cardiac surgery, PE, or trauma and is postulated to involve autoimmune mechanisms. The pain at presentation is similar to that of early pericarditis, but symptoms are often more systemic and include fever, leukocytosis, and polyserositis. In the era of rapid reperfusion therapy, the incidence of Dressler's syndrome has diminished.

Therapy of early and late pericarditis is similar and includes selected anti-inflammatory agents. The therapy of choice is aspirin, at high doses of up to 650 mg four times daily. Colchicine at doses up to 1.2 mg per day can be added for refractory pain. Nonsteroidal anti-inflammatory agents (NSAIDs), such as indomethacin or naproxen, are effective, but are best avoided. NSAIDs may contribute to infarct expansion and aneurysm formation, cause coronary vasocontriction, and adversely affect renal function. In addition, ibuprofen can reduce the antiplatelet effect of aspirin.[18] Similar to noninfarct-related pericarditis, corticosteroids should also be resisted as first-choice agents, since they frequently contribute to a transition from acute to chronic pericarditis.

A **pericardial effusion** is often seen with after an MI. These may be seen accompanying clinical pericarditis, but often occur in isolation. These effusions are typically small, resolve spontaneously, and require no follow-up imaging. However, in a subset of patients with clinical evidence of pericarditis accompanied by pericardial effusion, a follow-up echocardiogram is warranted, to forestall an emergency presentation with pericardial tamponade.

Arrhythmic complications of ACS

Bradyarrhythmias

Bradycardia and heart block following an acute coronary syndrome typically occur either because of exaggerated vagal tone, or due to the ischemia/infarction of the actual conduction tissue. Sinus bradycardia and varying degrees of AV block are often seen in *inferior* and *posterior MI* due to increased vagal tone. On the other hand, in *anterior MI* conduction disturbances are caused by necrosis of the bundle of His and its branches.

Sinus bradycardia and AV block may be observed in the early period of an inferior myocardial infarction. These vagally mediated bradycardias are often transient, and initially tend to respond to anticholinergic action of atropine. In the 24–72 hours following symptom onset, AV conduction delay may be caused by tissue edema (in addition to vagal tone) and is therefore less responsive to atropine. Second-degree heart block can occur either at the level of the AV node or below the node at the level of the His bundle. This differentiation is important, because it dictates an approach to therapy (Table 6.4).

Table 6.4 Differentiating the site of AV block in acute coronary syndrome

Site of block	AV node	Below node
Typical infarct location	• Inferior or posterior	• Anteroseptal
Usual mechanism	• Increased vagal tone	• Ischemia of septal perforator branches
ECG findings	• First-degree AV delay • Type 1 second-degree AV block (Mobitz I; Wenkebach)	• Type 2 second-degree AV block (Mobitz II) • Complete heart block
Characteristic ventricular escape	• Stable • Originates from proximal His bundle • Rate usually >40 bpm • Narrow QRS, resembling that during sinus rhythm	• Unstable • Originates in bundles of His or ventricular myocardium • Rate usually <40 bpm • Wide QRS

Continued

Table 6.4 Continued

Site of block	AV node	Below node
Prognosis	• Probably no increase in mortality	• Increased mortality as marker of larger infarction
Vagal maneuvers	• Block gets worse as sinus rate slows • Block improves with faster HR	• Block can improve with slower sinus rate
Tx	• Observation; atropine if ischemia or symptoms are present • Typically resolves • Rarely requires PPM	• Temporary transvenous pacemaker in most cases • Often requires a permanent pacemaker

The decision to place a temporary pacemaker in the setting of acute MI is affected by the nature of the conduction defect (Table 6.4) and the overall clinical assessment of the patient. The ACC/AHA guidelines for placement of a temporary transvenous pacemaker are listed in Table 6.5.

Table 6.5 A summary of the ACC/AHA guidelines: recommendations for temporary transvenous pacing in acute myocardial infarction

Class I

1 Asystole
2 Symptomatic bradycardia (includes sinus bradycardia with hypotension and type I second-degree AV block with hypotension not responsive to atropine)
3 Bilateral bundle branch block (alternating BBB or RBBB with alternating LAFB/ LPFB)
4 New or indeterminate-age bifascicular block (RBBB with LAFB or LPFB, or LBBB) with first-degree AV block
5 Mobitz type II second-degree AV block

Class IIa

1 RBBB and LAFB or LPFB (new or indeterminate)
2 RBBB with first-degree AV block
3 LBBB, new or indeterminate
4 Incessant ventricular tachycardia, for atrial or ventricular overdrive pacing
5 Recurrent sinus pauses (>3 seconds) not responsive to atropine

Continued

Class IIb

1 Bifascicular block of indeterminate age

2 New or indeterminate-age isolated RBBB

Class III

1 First-degree heart block

2 Type I second-degree AV block with normal hemodynamics

3 Accelerated idioventricular rhythm

4 BBB or fascicular block known to exist before AMI

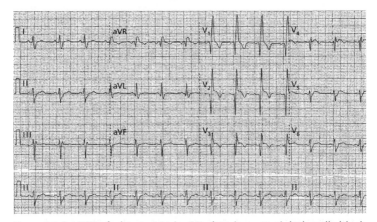

Figure 6.6 An ECG of a large anterior MI, showing new right bundle block and left anterior fascicular block. Note deep Q waves in leads V_1–V_3, with residual ST-segment elevations in leads V_1–V_4. Coronary angiography demonstrated a thrombotic occlusion of the proximal left anterior descending artery (image courtesy of John V. Wylie, M.D.).

As mentioned previously, many episodes of bradycardia and conduction abnormalities after an MI are transient, albeit occasionally symptomatic, phenomena, which resolve within hours to days of an acute ischemic insult. Nevertheless, a selected group of patients with extensive damage to the conduction system will require implantation of a *permanent* pacemaker. The ACC/AHA guidelines for permanent pacing after MI are outlined in Table 6.6.

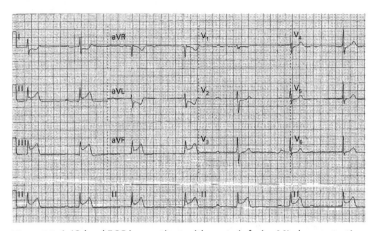

Figure 6.7 A 12-lead ECG in a patient with acute inferior MI, demonstrating complete heart block (image courtesy of John V. Wylie, M.D.).

Table 6.6 A summary of the ACC/AHA guidelines: permanent pacing after the acute phase of myocardial infarction (MI)

Class I
- Persistent second-degree AV block in the His–Purkinje system with bilateral bundle branch block
- Third-degree AV block within or below the His–Purkinje system
- Transient second- or third-degree infranodal AV block and associated bundle branch block; if the site of the block is uncertain, an electrophysiological study may be necessary
- Persistent and symptomatic second- or third-degree AV block

Class IIb
- Persistent second- or third-degree AV block at the AV node level

Class III
There is evidence that permanent pacing after the acute phase of MI is not useful and may be harmful in the following settings:
- Transient AV block in the absence of intraventricular conduction defects
- Transient AV block in the presence of isolated left anterior fascicular block
- Acquired left anterior fascicular block in the absence of AV block
- Persistent first-degree AV block in the presence of bundle branch block that is old or age-indeterminate

Atrial fibrillation

Atrial fibrillation is a common arrhythmia during and immediately following STEMI, occurring about 5–10% of the time. This is because many of the risk factors for STEMI, such as hypertension, obesity, and diabetes, are also the substrate for atrial fibrillation. Furthermore, the high catecholamine state and elevation of left atrial pressure in STEMI act as triggers for atrial fibrillation. An important consideration in atrial fibrillation is that rapid heart rates can increase myocardial ischemia and decrease cardiac output, thereby making early cardioversion an attractive option.

Ventricular tachycardia and fibrillation

Management of ventricular arrhythmias occurring late (>30 days) following ACS, as well as general issues of risk stratification for sudden cardiac death following ACS are discussed separately in Chapter 7.

Ventricular tachyarrhythmias occurring during and early following acute MI are the leading cause of death in ACS prior to hospital presentation. Indeed, in the contemporary era, sustained ventricular tachycardia (VT) and ventricular fibrillation (VF) complicate 10% of STEMI and 2.5% of NSTEACS presentation, with the majority occurring in the first 48 hours.[19,20] Patients with sustained VT are frequently symptomatic—both from hemodynamic effects of AV dissociation and from inefficient LV contraction, and therefore immediate therapy with synchronized cardioversion (defibrillation for VF) is required. Patients with well-tolerated sustained VT may be treated pharmacologically. Infrequently, recurrent episodes of sustained VT or VF occur after ACS, without underlying ischemia/reinfarction. This is known as **electrical storm**, and it presents a major therapeutic challenge. Aggressive beta adrenergic blockade and VT ablation have been used in electrical storm with some success.[21]

Isolated ventricular premature beats (VPB) and nonsustained ventricular tachycardia (NSVT) are ubiquitous after ACS. When they occur in the first 72 hours following ACS, these are no longer thought to portend a poor prognosis, and do not require primary antiarrhythmic treatment. Any increase in frequency of ventricular arrhythmia early after ACS should prompt a search for recurrent myocardial ischemia. The latter is addressed with standard antiischemic therapy and revascularization, when appropriate.

Accelerated idioventricular rhythm (AIVR) is a related arrhythmia seen in the early postinfarction period. It is a regular wide complex rhythm at rates <120 bpm, frequently associated with successful reperfusion of the infarct-related artery (Figure 6.8). AIVR is usually asymptomatic, terminates spontaneously, and is not associated with sustained VT/VF. Antiarrhythmic therapy for AIVR is not necessary, and may in fact become deleterious through suppression of the ventricular escape mechanism in AIVR.

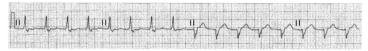

Figure 6.8 Accelerated idioventricular rhythm (AIVR) 2 hours following successful reperfusion of an anterior STEMI.

Complications involving bleeding

Significant bleeding which necessitates red blood cell transfusion complicates approximately 1 in 10 cases of thrombolysis for STEMI.[22] The most dreaded bleeding complication of thrombolysis, however, is intracranial hemorrhage (ICH). This is seen in less than 1% of thrombolysis, but the case fatality rate for ICH after thrombolysis is high, approaching 60%. The risk of ICH after thrombolysis depends on patient comorbidities, on the thrombolytic agent used, and on comcomitant antithrombotic therapy. A simple risk score was developed by the Cooperative Cardiovascular Project to predict the risk of ICH, with the highest group having a rate of intracranial bleeding that exceeds 4% (Table 6.7).[23]

Management of ICH includes an immediate noncontrast computed tomography scan of the brain to confirm bleeding and to assess its extent and distribution. Anticoagulant and antithrombin therapy is stopped and baseline laboratory assessment of hemoglobin, platelet count, and

Table 6.7 The Cooperative Cardiovascular Project risk model for intracranial hemorrhage with thrombolytic therapy (data from Brass et al.[23])

Risk factors	Number of risk factors	Rate of intracranial hemorrhage
Age ≥75 years		
Black race	0 or 1	0.69%
Female gender	2	1.02%
Prior history of stroke	3	1.63%
Systolic blood pressure ≥ 160 mmHg	4	2.49%
Weight ≤65 kg for women or ≤80 kg for men	≥5	4.11%
INR >4 or PT >24 seconds		
Use of alteplase (versus other thrombolytic agents)		

coagulation factors is performed. Pharmacologic effects of antithrombotic therapy are reversed by administration of fresh frozen plasma, cryoprecipitate, and a platelet transfusion. Emergency neurologic and neurosurgical consultations are obtained and general measures to reduce intracranial pressure are instituted. Endotracheal intubation may become necessary to maintain low-to-normal carbon dioxide tension, and craniotomy to reduce intracranial pressure should not be delayed.

Complications of percutaneous coronary intervention

Since the introduction of diagnostic left heart catheterization in the early 1950s and PCI in the late 1970s, both procedures have had remarkable improvements in their safety.[24,25] For diagnostic catheterization, the rate of death is <0.1% and is seen primarily in patients with severe comorbidities such as CHF, left main disease, critical AS, and severe renal disease. The risks are slightly higher in the setting of acute coronary syndrome and urgent catheterization, but are generally outweighed by the benefits of revascularization. Table 6.8 lists the

Table 6.8 Complications of coronary angiography and percutaneous coronary intervention

Cardiac catheterization and PCI complication	Definition	Risk factors	Presentation and diagnostic testing	Prevention	Treatment
Hematoma	• Blood collection at site of arterial access	• Age • Female • Renal disease • Peripheral arterial disease • Obesity	• Physical examination • Ultrasound may be necessary to exclude AV fistula or pseudo-aneurysm	• Meticulous access technique • Awareness of small hematoma formation during case in order to apply pressure and prevent extension	• Direct pressure above site of bleeding • Pressure dressing
AV fistula	• Connection between the artery and vein	• Similar to those with hematoma	• Suspected by presence of new continuous bruit at the access site • Especially if continuous; ultrasound to confirm	• Meticulous access technique • Arterial puncture above the bifurcation of superficial femoral artery and profunda femoris	• Small AV fistulae may close spontaneously • Large AV fistulae need surgical repair
Pseudoaneurysm	A contained hematoma with flow in and out of the vessel	• Similar to those with hematoma	• Ultrasound	• Meticulous access technique • Inadequate duration of arterial compression following sheath removal	• Small pseudoaneurysms (<2 cm) can be closed by ultrasound-guided injection of thrombin • Larger pseudoaneurysms require surgical repair

Retroperitoneal bleeding	• Bleeding at access site above the inguinal ligament which causes blood to accumulate in RP	• Similar to those with hematoma	• Presents as ipsilateral back pain • Tachycardia and hypotension may complicate large RP bleed • Abdominal/pelvic computed tomography	• Meticulous access technique • Arterial puncture above the bifurcation of superficial femoral artery and profunda femoris	• Observation, serial imaging • May require blood transfusion and reversal of anticoagulation
Access site thrombosis	• Thrombus formation at site of sheath placement, causing vascular compromise	• Small vessel • Peripheral vascular disease • Diabetes • Large sheath • Intraaortic balloon pump	• Presents as the triad of pain, pallor, and poikilothermia in the leg • Prolonged vascular compromise results in paresthesia and paralysis • Suspected by decreased pulses in the affected extremity • Confirmed with vascular ultrasound	• Use of smallest sheath possible • Prompt removal of sheath • Anticoagulation with IABP	• Anticoagulation • Catheter-based thrombectomy • Surgery

Continued

Table 6.8 Continued

Cardiac catheterization and PCI complication	Definition	Risk factors	Presentation and diagnostic testing	Prevention	Treatment
Stroke	• May result from embolism of *de novo* platelet thrombus or fragments of displaced calcium from catheter manipulation	• Age, pvd, poor technique • Crossing of a calcified stenotic aortic valve	• New neurologic deficit following angiography/PCI (or often subclinical) • Peripheral embolization can present with livedo reticularis (cholesterol embolism syndrome) • Renal embolization can present with renal failure and peripheral eosinophilia	• Catheter exchange below the diaphragm to prevent cerebral emboli • Upper extremity access in cases of known mobile descending aortic plaque • Avoidance of unnecessary crossing of calcified aortic valve	• Supportive
Renal failure	• May be due to: – cholesterol emboli	• Baseline renal dysfunction • Dehydration • Diabetes mellitus	• Serum creatinine • Urine sediment	• Minimization of contrast load • Use of iso-osmolar contrast agent	• Supportive • Minimize hypotension

	– contrast nephropathy – prolonged hypotension	• Large contrast load		• N-acetylcysteine before and after catheterization • Intravenous hydration and sodium bicarbonate infusion prior to catheterization	• Supportive
Radiation burn	• Usually presents days to weeks following exposure	• radiation load (often required in obese patients)	• Skin irritation, ulceration, usually on the back or chest	• Decrease radiation exposure • Use of varied angiography projections during the case	
Contrast allergy	• Anaphylaxis • Delayed-type hypersensitivity	• Prior contrast reaction • Possible association with allergy to shellfish	• Examination	• Patients with known allergy to contrast should be pretreated with steroids and histamine blockers	• Epinephrine for anaphylaxis • Steroids and antihistamines for delayed hypersensitivity

common complications of PCI and suggests specific treatment.

References

1. Rogers WJ, Canto JG, Lambrew CT, *et al*. Temporal trends in the treatment of over 1.5 million patients with myocardial infarction in the US from 1990 through 1999: the National Registry of Myocardial Infarction 1, 2 and 3. *J Am Coll Cardiol* 2000; 36: 2056–63.
2. Holmes Dr, Jr., Berger PB, Hochman JS, *et al*. Cardiogenic shock in patients with acute ischemic syndromes with and without ST-segment elevation. *Circulation* 1999; 100: 2067–73.
3. Jeger RV, Radovanovic D, Hunziker PR, *et al*. Ten-year trends in the incidence and treatment of cardiogenic shock. *Ann Intern Med* 2008; 149: 618–26.
4. Hochman JS, Boland J, Sleeper LA, *et al*. Current spectrum of cardiogenic shock and effect of early revascularization on mortality. Results of an International Registry. SHOCK Registry Investigators. *Circulation* 1995; 91: 873–81.
5. Killip T, 3rd, Kimball JT. Treatment of myocardial infarction in a coronary care unit. A two year experience with 250 patients. *Am J Cardiol* 1967; 20: 457–64.
6. Bengtson JR, Kaplan AJ, Pieper KS, *et al*. Prognosis in cardiogenic shock after acute myocardial infarction in the interventional era. *J Am Coll Cardiol* 1992; 20: 1482–9.
7. Zimetbaum PJ, Josephson ME. Use of the electrocardiogram in acute myocardial infarction. *N Engl J Med* 2003; 348: 933–40.
8. Zehender M, Kasper W, Kauder E, *et al*. Right ventricular infarction as an independent predictor of prognosis after acute inferior myocardial infarction. *N Engl J Med* 1993; 328: 981–8.
9. Ferrario M, Poli A, Previtali M, *et al*. Hemodynamics of volume loading compared with dobutamine in severe right ventricular infarction. *Am J Cardiol* 1994; 74: 329–33.
10. Mehta SR, Eikelboom JW, Natarajan MK, *et al*. Impact of right ventricular involvement on mortality and morbidity in patients with inferior myocardial infarction. *J Am Coll Cardiol* 2001; 37: 37–43.
11. Cabin HS, Roberts WC. Left ventricular aneurysm, intraaneurysmal thrombus and systemic embolus in coronary heart disease. *Chest* 1980; 77: 586–90.
12. Turpie AG, Robinson JG, Doyle DJ, *et al*. Comparison of high-dose with low-dose subcutaneous heparin to prevent left ventricular mural thrombosis in patients with acute transmural anterior myocardial infarction. *N Engl J Med* 1989; 320: 352–7.

13. Vaitkus PT, Barnathan ES. Embolic potential, prevention and management of mural thrombus complicating anterior myocardial infarction: a meta-analysis. *J Am Coll Cardiol* 1993; 22: 1004–9.

14. Antman EM, Hand M, Armstrong PW, *et al*. 2007 focused update of the ACC/AHA 2004 guidelines for the management of patients with ST-elevation myocardial infarction: a report of the American College of Cardiology/American Heart Association Task Force on Practice Guidelines. *J Am Coll Cardiol* 2008; 51: 210–47.

15. Antman EM, Anbe DT, Armstrong PW, *et al*. ACC/AHA guidelines for the management of patients with ST-elevation myocardial infarction: a report of the American College of Cardiology/American Heart Association Task Force on Practice Guidelines (Committee to Revise the 1999 Guidelines for the Management of Patients with Acute Myocardial Infarction). *Circulation* 2004; 110: e82–e292.

16. Dor V, Sabatier M, Montiglio F, Rossi P, Toso A, Di Donato M. Results of nonguided subtotal endocardiectomy associated with left ventricular reconstruction in patients with ischemic ventricular arrhythmias. *J Thorac Cardiovasc Surg* 1994; 107: 1301–7; discussion 1307–8.

17. Yeo TC, Malouf JF, Oh JK, Seward JB. Clinical profile and outcome in 52 patients with cardiac pseudoaneurysm. *Ann Intern Med* 1998; 128: 299–305.

18. Catella-Lawson F, Reilly MP, Kapoor SC, *et al*. Cyclooxygenase inhibitors and the antiplatelet effects of aspirin. *N Engl J Med* 2001; 345: 1809–17.

19. Newby KH, Thompson T, Stebbins A, Topol EJ, Califf RM, Natale A. Sustained ventricular arrhythmias in patients receiving thrombolytic therapy: incidence and outcomes. The GUSTO Investigators. *Circulation* 1998; 98: 2567–73.

20. Al-Khatib SM, Granger CB, Huang Y, *et al*. Sustained ventricular arrhythmias among patients with acute coronary syndromes with no ST-segment elevation: incidence, predictors, and outcomes. *Circulation* 2002; 106: 309–12.

21. Nademanee K, Taylor R, Bailey WE, Rieders DE, Kosar EM. Treating electrical storm : sympathetic blockade versus advanced cardiac life support-guided therapy. *Circulation* 2000; 102: 742–7.

22. Berkowitz SD, Granger CB, Pieper KS, *et al*. Incidence and predictors of bleeding after contemporary thrombolytic therapy for myocardial infarction. The Global Utilization of Streptokinase and Tissue Plasminogen activator for Occluded coronary arteries (GUSTO) I Investigators. *Circulation* 1997; 95: 2508–16.

23. Brass LM, Lichtman JH, Wang Y, Gurwitz JH, Radford MJ, Krumholz HM. Intracranial hemorrhage associated with thrombolytic therapy for elderly patients with acute myocardial infarction: results from the Cooperative Cardiovascular Project. *Stroke* 2000; 31: 1802–11.

24. Yang EH, Gumina RJ, Lennon RJ, Holmes DR, Jr., Rihal CS, Singh M. Emergency coronary artery bypass surgery for percutaneous coronary interventions: changes in the incidence, clinical characteristics, and indications from 1979 to 2003. *J Am Coll Cardiol* 2005; 46: 2004–9.

25. Anderson HV, Shaw RE, Brindis RG, *et al.* A contemporary overview of percutaneous coronary interventions. The American College of Cardiology–National Cardiovascular Data Registry (ACC–NCDR). *J Am Coll Cardiol* 2002; 39: 1096–103.

CHAPTER 7

Post-hospitalization care of patients with acute coronary syndrome

Jersey Chen and Eli V. Gelfand

Introduction

Patients with ACS are at high risk for recurrent evensts. Long-term data from the Olmstead County, MN epidemiologic study from 1979 to 1998 demonstrate that within 3 years after acute MI, over 40% of patients suffer recurrent MI or unstable angina, and 6% suffer sudden cardiac death.[1] The goal of secondary prevention is to reduce death and recurrent ischemic events in these high-risk patients.

Which risk factors should we target for secondary prevention after ACS? Understanding and targeting the risk factors most likely to affect the risk of recurrent events may be the most effective methods of initiating secondary prevention (Figure 7.1).

Pharmacologic measures

Aspirin

Aspirin substantially reduces the risk of cardiovascular events after MI through its antiplatelet properties. A meta-analysis of 12 randomized clinical trials of 18,788 patients with prior MI from the Antiplatelet Trialists' Collaboration demonstrated a 25% relative risk reduction for the risk of recurrent MI, stroke, or CV death with an effective range

Management of Acute Coronary Syndromes   Eli V. Gelfand and Christopher P. Cannon
© 2009 John Wiley & Sons, Ltd

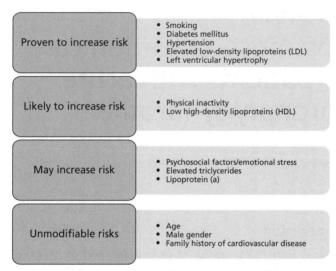

Figure 7.1 A risk factor classification for coronary heart disease.

from 75 to 325 mg daily (an absolute risk reduction of 36 events per 1,000 patients treated over an average of 27 months). The Antiplatelet Trialists' Collaboration did not demonstrate excess extracranial bleeding with dosages > 162 mg/d, although other studies suggest higher bleeding events with dosages > 100 or 162 mg/d (CURE and BRAVO, respectively). The 2006 ACC/AHA secondary prevention guidelines recommend indefinite use of aspirin 75–162 mg daily; a 325 mg daily dose is not uncommon in the U.S.

Patients with aspirin allergy may undergo aspirin desensitization therapy in an appropriately monitored clinical setting (see the Appendix). Alternatively, clopidogrel, ticlopidine, or warfarin can be used in aspirin-allergic patients (discussed below).

Clopidogrel

Several studies have assessed the optimal dose and duration of clopidogrel therapy after ACS, with or without stenting (Table 7.1). There is little controversy in that clopidogrel is an effective *alternative* to aspirin monotherapy in patients with a true aspirin allergy. The addition of clopidogrel to aspirin is associated with an increased risk of bleeding, but as data below show, improves outcomes following ACS.

Table 7.1 Major RCTs of clopidogrel after ACS

Study	Population	n	Dose/titration	Effectiveness
CAPRIE	MI, CVA, PAD	19,185	Clopidogrel 75 mg vs. aspirin 325 mg	9.8% vs. 10.64% for MI, CVA, death; $p = 0.045$
CURE	ACS within 24 hours	12,562	Clopidogrel 300 mg load, then 75 mg daily) in addition to aspirin for 3–12 months	9.3% in the PLAVIX group and 11.4%, for MI, CVA, death, $p < 0.001$
PCI-CURE	ACS within 24 hours undergoing PCI	2,658	Clopidogrel 300 mg load, then 75 mg daily × mean 8 months vs. placebo load and open label clopidogrel 75 mg × 4 weeks after PCI	4.5% vs. 6.4% for death, MI, target vessel revascularization in 30 days, $p = 0.03$
CLARITY-TIMI28	STEMI	3,491	Clopidogrel 300 mg load then 75 mg × 30 days vs. placebo	11.6% vs. 14.1% for CV death, MI, recurrent ischemia (%), $p < 0.03$
CREDO	Elective PCI (34% prior MI)	2,116	Clopidogrel 300 mg load then 75 mg—1 year vs. 75 mg × 30 d	8.5% vs. 11.5% for MI, CVA, death at 1 year, $p = 0.02$
CHARISMA	CAD, CVA/TIA, PAD or multiple risk factors for CVD	15,603	Clopidogrel 75 mg plus ASA 75–162 mg daily vs. placebo plus ASA 75–162 mg daily	6.8% vs. 7.3% in MI, CVA, death at 42 months, $p = 0.22$ (subgroup with established CVD, 6.9% vs. 7.9% for MI, CVA, death, $p = 0.046$)

The CAPRIE trial demonstrated that clopidogrel 75 mg daily was minimally superior to aspirin 325 mg daily for the secondary prevention of MI stroke or vascular death in patients with prior MI, stroke, or PAD.[2] The CURE study found that in patients with ACS, the addition of clopidogrel (300 mg load, followed by 75 mg once daily for 3–12 months (mean, 9 months) reduced the composite outcome of CV death, MI, or stroke compared with aspirin alone.[3]

The PCI-CURE study examined a subgroup of patients from CURE, who underwent PCI. The study examined whether pretreatment with clopidogrel 300 mg followed by long-term therapy after PCI for a mean of 9 months was superior to a strategy of no pretreatment and only short-term clopidogrel therapy for 4 weeks after PCI. All patients received aspirin in addition to the study drug. A primary endpoint of cardiovascular death, MI, or urgent target vessel revascularization at 30 days after PCI was reached by 4.5% patients in the clopidogrel group, compared with 6.4% in the placebo group, a 30% relative risk reduction.[4]

While not an ACS patient-specific trial, CREDO examined whether extending clopidogrel treatment to 1 year after PCI was effective. All patients received a loading dose of clopidogrel 300 mg 24 hours before PCI, followed by either 28 days or 1 year of maintenance therapy. The principal result of CREDO was a 26.9% relative risk reduction (8.5% vs. 11.5%) in the primary endpoint of death, MI, or stroke among patients on clopidogrel for 1 year following PCI versus those on placebo treatment.[5]

The CHARISMA trial examined long-term clopidogrel in patients with stable vascular disease (outside of ACS) or multiple risk factors for vascular events. Patients were randomized to clopidogrel 75 mg plus or placebo plus low-dose aspirin for a median of 28 months. All patients received low-dose aspirin 75–162 mg. There was no difference in primary event rate (MI, stroke, or CV death) with clopidogrel 6.8% with clopidogrel plus aspirin and 7.3% with placebo plus aspirin (relative risk, 0.93). In a subgroup with established vascular disease (32% with prior MI), there was a reduction in primary outcome of 6.9% versus 7.9% (relative risk, 0.88). However, in a subgroup of patients with multiple risk factors,

Box 7.1 Antiplatelet therapy

- Start aspirin 75–162 mg/d and continue indefinitely in all patients unless contraindicated.
- For patients undergoing CABG, start aspirin within 48 hours after surgery to reduce saphenous vein graft closure.
- Start and continue clopidogrel 75 mg/d in combination with aspirin for up to 12 months in patients after ACS or percutaneous coronary intervention with stent placement:
  - $\geq$1 month for bare metal stent;
  - $\geq$3 months for sirolimus-, zotarolimus-, and everolimus-eluting stents (Cypher, Endeavor, Xience);
  - $\geq$6 months for aclitaxel-eluting stent (Taxus).
- Administer higher-dose aspirin at 325 mg/d after PCI with stent placement for patients who have undergone percutaneous coronary intervention with stent for 1 month for bare metal stent, 3 months for sirolimus-eluting stent, and 6 months for paclitaxel-eluting stent.

there was a significant increase in CV death and a trend towards increased primary endpoint with clopidogrel.[6]

Beta adrenergic blockade

Beta-blockers reduce mortality after ACS by reducing the incidence of fatal ventricular tachyarrhythmias and attenuating the effects of adverse cardiac remodeling in patients with left ventricular systolic dysfunction. Data from multiple randomized controlled trials have demonstrated that long-term beta-blockers should be administered to all patients who are able to tolerate therapy (Table 7.2). A meta-analysis of trials for secondary prevention, involving 54,234 patients, suggested a 23% decrease in mortality. In the meta-analysis, 42 patients needed to be treated with beta-blockers over 2 years to save one life.[7] Recently a new beta-blocker, nebivolol, has been approved for treatment of hypertension, but studies have not confirmed its efficacy in ACS.

Table 7.2 Major randomized controlled trials of beta-blockers after ACS

Study	Population	n (f/u)	Dose/titration	Effectiveness
BHAT	5–21 days post-MI	3,837 (24 months)	propranolol 180–240 mg/d	7.2% vs. 9.8%— CAD death
Norwegian Timolol Study	7–28 days post-MI	1,884 (17 months)	timolol 10 mg bid	7.7% vs. 13.9%— CAD death
Göteborg metoprolol trial	Acute MI	1,395 (90 days)	metoprolol 15 mg IV then 200 mg/d × 90 days	8.9% vs. 5.7%— death
ISIS-1	Acute MI in CCU	16,027 (7 days)	atenolol 5–10 mg IV, then 100 mg/d × 7 days	3.9% vs. 4.6%— vascular death

It is the ACC/AHA recommendation that beta-blocker therapy should be continued indefinitely in all patients able to tolerate it.

In post-infarct patients with heart failure from left ventricular dysfunction, beta-blockers should be initiated cautiously and titrated slowly to goal dosage. The specific agents and goal dosages of beta-blockers in hemodynamically stable heart failure patients should preferably reflect those evaluated by the major RCTs (Table 7.3). Carvedilol, bisoprolol, and extended-release metoprolol (metoprolol succinate) are currently FDA-approved for the treatment of heart failure.

Table 7.3 Major RCTs of beta-blockers after MI and heart failure with depressed LVEF

Study	Population	n	Dose/titration	Effectiveness
MERIT-HF	NYHA class II to IV HF and LVEF < 40% (48% post-MI)	3,991	Metoprolol XL 12.5–25 mg/d, titrate to 200 mg/d (mean 159 mg/d)	7.2% vs. 11% all-cause mortality over median 1 year
U.S. Carvedilol HF Study Group	HF and LVEF ≤ 35% (67% ischemic etiology)	1,094	Carvedilol 6.25 mg bid titrate to 25 mg bid	3.2% vs. 7.8% all-cause mortality over 6.5 months

Continued

Study	Population	n	Dose/titration	Effectiveness
CAPRICORN	Post-MI and LVEF ≤ 40%	1,959	Carvedilol 6.25 mg/d, titrate to 25 mg bid	11.7% vs. 15.5% all-cause morality over mean 1.3 years
CIBIS II	NYHA class III or IV HF and LVEF ≤ 35% (50% ischemic etiology)	2,647	Bisoprolol 1.25 mg/d titrate to 10 mg/d	11.8% vs. 17.3% all-cause death over 1.4 years

Box 7.2 Beta adrenergic blockade for secondary prevention

- Start and continue indefinitely in all patients who have had myocardial infarction, acute coronary syndrome, or left ventricular dysfunction with or without heart failure symptoms, unless contraindicated.
- Consider chronic therapy for all other patients with coronary or other vascular disease or diabetes unless contraindicated.

Renin–angiotensin–aldosterone inhibitors

Angiotensin-converting enzyme inhibitor therapy

Multiple RCTs have demonstrated the efficacy of angiotensin-converting enzyme (ACE) inhibitors for secondary prevention (Table 7.4). The greatest benefit has been observed for patients at higher risk, particularly those with low LVEF or large and anterior infarctions. Because of their beneficial effects in hypertension, diabetes, or chronic renal insufficiency, ACE inhibitors are strongly recommended in patients with these conditions. ACE inhibitors should be considered in all other post-ACS patients. The AIRE Extension study demonstrated sustained benefit out to 5 years of ramipril versus placebo post MI[8] (Figure 7.2).

Table 7.4 Major RCTs of ACE inhibitors after ACS

Study	Population	n	Dose/titration	Effectiveness
SAVE	Post-AMI (3–16 days) with asymptomatic LVEF ≤ 40% I	2,231	Captopril 12.5 mg/d to 25 mg/tid at d/c, 50 mg/tid max	(188/1,115, 244/1,116) CV death at 42 m
AIRE	Post-AMI (3–10 days) with symptomatic HF	2,006	Ramapril 5 mg bid	17% vs. 23% all-cause death at 15 months
TRACE	Post-AMI (3–17 days) with LVEF < 35%	1,749	Trandalopril 1 mg/d to 2 mg/d at day 2, to 4 mg at week 2	35.7% vs. 42.3% all-cause death at 24–50 months
SOLVD	Hospitalized chronic HF (66% post MI)	2,569	Enalapril 2.5–5 mg bid to max 10 mg bid	35.2% vs. 39.7% all-cause death at 41.4 months
EUROPA	Stable CAD without HF (65% prior MI)	12,218	Perindopril 4 mg/d × 2 weeks run-in, then 8 mg/d	8.0% vs. 9.9%, CV death, MI, cardiac arrest at 4.2 years
HOPE	CVD or DM + risk factors without low LVEF or HF (80% prior MI)	9,297	Ramapril 2.5, 5, then 10 mg/d	14.0% vs. 17.8%, CV death, MI, stroke at 5 years
PEACE	CAD with LVEF > 40% without DM or HF (55% prior MI)	8,290	Trandolapril 2 mg/d × 6 months then 4 mg/d	21.9% vs. 22.5% ($p = 0.43$) CV death, MI, revascularization at 4.8 years

ACE inhibitors may be optional in patients at the lowest risk with well-controlled risk factors and coronary revascularization. The PEACE trial failed to find a benefit for trandolapril in CAD patients with normal LVEF without DM or HF and well-controlled lipid levels on statin therapy.[9] Despite the results of this trial and the associated ACC/AHA recommendations, we feel that given the presumed vascular endothelial dysfunction in the vast majority of patients with ACS, it is difficult to find a "low-enough risk" group of patients in whom ACE inhibitors should be withheld.

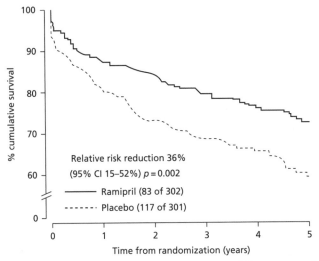

Figure 7.2 Five-year survival in the AIRE Extension trial (from Tognoni and Franzosi[8]).

Box 7.3 Antagonism of the renin–angiotensin–aldosterone axis in secondary prevention

ACE inhibitors (ACE-I)
- All patients with LVEF ≤ 40% and those with hypertension, diabetes, or chronic kidney disease, unless contraindicated.
- *Consider* for all patients post-ACS.
- Optional in lower-risk patients with normal LVEF in whom cardiovascular risk factors are well controlled and revascularization has been performed.

Angiotensin receptor blockers
- Use in patients who intolerant of ACE-I, and:
  - have clinical heart failure, or
  - have had a MI with LVEF ≤ 40%.
- *Consider* in other patients who are ACE-I intolerant.
- *Consider* use in combination with ACE-I systolic-dysfunction heart failure.

Box 7.3 Continued

Aldosterone blockers
- Post-myocardial infarction patients, without significant renal dysfunction or hyperkalemia, who are already receiving therapeutic doses of an ACE inhibitor and beta-blocker, and have LVEF ≤ 40% and at least one of the following:
  - diabetes mellitus;
  - clinical evidence of heart failure.

Angiotensin receptor blocker therapy

The VALIANT, ELITE II, and CHARM-Alternative studies demonstrated that angiotensin receptor blockers (ARB) valsartan or candesartan appear to be equivalent to ACE inhibitors in post-MI patients with heart failure and low LVEF.[10–12] However, the OPTIMAAL trial of losartan 50 mg/d compared with captopril 50 mg/tid in patients with HF or left-ventricular dysfunction after MI demonstrated that a nonsignificant difference in total mortality was seen in favor of captopril.[13] The ACC/AHA guidelines recommend the use of ARBs in patients who are unable to tolerate ACE inhibitors.

Two studies examined combination therapy of ACE inhibitors and ARBs in heart failure patients. The CHARM-Added trial found that the addition of candesartan to ACE inhibitors reduced the composite outcome of CV death or HF hospitalization compared with ACE inhibitors alone.[14] The VALIANT study found that the addition of valsartan to captopril was equivalent for all-cause mortality, although more adverse effects of hypotension and renal dysfunction were reported.[10] In the 2007 AHA/ACC UA/NSTEMI guideline revision, the combination of an ACE inhibitor and ARB is a class IIb recommendation for patients with persistent symptomatic HF and LVEF < 40%, despite conventional therapy including either an ACE inhibitor or ARB alone (Table 7.5). In the 2006 AHA/ACC secondary prevention guidelines, combination therapy of

ACE inhibitor and ARB in patients with LV systolic dysfunction is a level Ib recommendation. The 2004 AHA/ACC STEMI guidelines state that combination therapy with candesartan (preferred) or valsartan can be considered for patients after STEMI with symptomatic HF and LVEF < 40% in patients without significant renal dysfunction or hyperkalemia.

Table 7.5 Major RCTs of ARBs alone or in combination with ACE inhibitors

Study	Population	n	Dose/titration	Effectiveness
VALIANT	AMI (5–10 days post MI) with HF failure or LVEF < 35%	14,703	Valsartan (up to 160 mg bid), captopril (up to 50 mg tid), or valsartan plus captopril (up to 80 mg bid and 50 mg tid, respectively)	• No significant difference in all-cause mortality 19.9% (valsartan) 19.5% (captopril) 19.3% (combination) at median 24.7 months • Combination therapy had more adverse events
ELITE-II	HF with LVEF ≤ 40%	3,152	Losartan 50 mg/d, captopril 50 mg tid	• No significant difference in all-cause mortality 11.7% (losartan) 10.4% (captopril)
Val-HeFT	HF and LVEF < 40%	5,010	Valsartan 40 mg bid titrate to 160 mg/d vs. placebo	• No significant difference in death 19.7% vs. 19.4% • Significant difference for death, HF, hospitalization, cardiac arrest, intravenous therapy 28.8% vs. 32.1%, over mean 23 months

Continued

Table 7.5 Continued

Study	Population	n	Dose/titration	Effectiveness
CHARM-Added	Chronic HF and LVEF ≤ 40% already taking ACE inhibitor, with or without beta-blocker	2,548	Candesartan 4 or 8 mg/d, titrate q2w to 32 mg/d	38% vs. 42% for CV death or HF hospitalization at median 41 months
OPTIMAAL	AMI with HF or LVEF < 35%	5,477	Losartan 12.5 mg/d titrate to 50 mg/d, or captopril 12.5 mg tid titrated to 50 mg tid	18% vs. 16% for death over mean follow-up of 2.7 years
CHARM-Alternative	Chronic HF and LVEF ≤ 40% unable to tolerate ACE inhibitor	2,028	Candesartan 4 or 8 mg/d, titrate to 32 mg/d	33% vs. 40% for CV death or HF hospitalization at median 33.7 m

Aldosterone blockade

Aldosterone blockade with spironolactone or eplerenone has been demonstrated to reduce all-cause mortality in patients with severe chronic systolic heart failure (including after ACS) and specifically within 2 weeks following acute MI (Table 7.6). The 2006 AHA/ACC secondary prevention guidelines recommend aldosterone blockade in patients with LVEF ≤ 40% with either HF or diabetes, and without renal dysfunction or hyperkalemia already no therapeutic dosages of ACE inhibitiors and beta-blockers. Mineralocorticoid receptor antagonists may attenuate adverse cardiac remodeling after a myocardial infarction regardless of the initial systolic ventricular function; however, data on clinical outcomes with their use in patients with preserved LVEF undergoing PCI

Table 7.6 Major RCTs of aldosterone antagonists for patients with HF and depressed LVEF

Study	Population	n	Dose/titration	Effectiveness
RALES	NYHA Class IV HF within 6 months and LVEF < 35%, treated with ACE inhibitors (55% ischemic HF)	1,663	Spironolactone 25mg/d titrate to 50mg/d if still symptomatic	All-cause mortality 35% vs. 46%
EPHESUS	AMI within 2 weeks with LVEF < 40% and HF	6,642	eplerenone 25 mg/d, man 50 mg/d	All-cause mortality 14.4% vs. 16.7% CV death and hospitalization 26.7% vs. 30%

are not yet available. In the EPHESUS trial, there was a substantial rate of serious hyperkalemia (5.5% vs. 3.9%), underscoring the need for close monitoring of serum potassium level.[15]

Lipid-lowering therapy

Therapy to lower LDL cholesterol

Multiple RCTs have demonstrated that **HMG-CoA reductase inhibitors (statins)** reduce CAD death and recurrent MI in post-ACS patients (Table 7.7). This benefit is throughout a wide range of pretreatment lipid levels. The PROVE-IT and MIRACL studies suggest that early high-dose statin therapy appears to confer additional benefit after MI.[16,17]

The NCEP/ATP III Update 2004 guidelines recommend persons with CAD to attain LDL of <100 mg/dl. The ACC/AHA guidelines recommend a goal LDL of <100, with further reduction to <70 as a reasonable goal. If LDL goal is not achieved with diet and statin therapy, additional options include adding niacin or fibrate therapy.

In the pre-statin era, the Coronary Drug Project of male patients after MI found that **niacin** was associated with an 11% reduction in mortality (52.0% vs. 58.2%) compared

Table 7.7 Major RCTs of statins

Study	Population	n	Dose/titration	Effectiveness
4S	Angina or MI with high cholesterol	4,444	Simvastatin 20, mg/d titrate to 10–40 mg/d	5.0% vs. 8.5% CAD death at 5.4 years
CARE	Post-MI (3–20 months) with average cholesterol	4,159	Pravastatin 40 mg/d	10.2% vs. 13.2% CAD death/MI at 5 years
LIPID	Post-MI (3–36 months) with wide range cholesterol	9,014	Pravastatin 40 mg/d	6.4% vs. 8.3% CAD death, 7.4% vs. 10.3% MI at 6.1 years
Heart Protection Study	CVD with wide range cholesterol	20,536	Pravastatin 40 mg/d	5.7% vs. 6.9% CAD death, 8.7% vs. 11.8% CAD events at 5 years
PROVE IT– TIMI 22	ACS within 10 days	4,162	Atorvastatin 80 mg/d vs. pravastatin 40 mg/d	22.4% vs. 26.3% for all-cause death, MI, UA, revascularization at least 30 days after, and stroke at 24 months
TNT	CAD with LDL < 130	10,001	Atorvastatin 80 mg vs. 10 mg/d	8.7% vs. 10.9% for CAD death, MI, cardiac arrest, or stroke at median 4.9 years
IDEAL	Prior MI	8,888	Atorvastatin 80 mg/d vs. simvastatin 20 mg/d	Nonsignificant difference (10.4% vs. 9.3%) for coronary death, MI, or cardiac arrest at median 4.8 years

Continued

Study	Population	n	Dose/titration	Effectiveness
A to Z (phase Z)	ACS	4,497	Simvastatin 40 mg/d × 1 month then 80 mg/d thereafter vs placebo × 4 months then simvastatin 20 mg/d	Nonsignificant trend 14.4% vs. 16.4% ($p = 0.14$) for cardiovascular death, MI, readmission for ACS, and stroke over 6–24 months
MIRACL	ACS (24–96 hours)	3,086	Atorvastatin 80 mg/d vs. placebo	14.8% vs. 17.4% ($p = 0.048$) for death, MI, cardiac arrest, and recurrent ischemia over 4 months

with placebo after 15 years of follow-up, but 9 years after the end of the trial.[18] No RCT data with clinical outcomes are available regarding additional benefit of niacin combined with statin therapy.

At the present time, ezetimide should be reserved solely for patients who are unable to achieve goal LDL levels on maximal tolerated dose of statin.

Therapy for low-HDL cholesterol or elevated triglycerides after MI

Post-MI patients with LDL cholesterol near goal who continue to have low-HDL (<40 mg/dl) cholesterol appear to benefit from treatment to raise HDL (Table 7.8). In this population, gemfibrozil has been demonstrated to reduce cardiac events in the VA-HIT study.[19] Prescription (not dietary supplement) niacin is another alternative.

If triglycerides are 200–499 mg/dl, the 2006 AHA/ACC guidelines recommend pharmacologic treatment to non-HDL level at least <130, with further reduction to <100 as is reasonable. If triglycerides are >500 mg/dl,

Table 7.8 Major RCTs of therapies for elevated HDL and triglyceride after MI

Study	Population	n	Dose/titration	Effectiveness
AFREGS	CAD with LDL < 160 and HDL < 40	143	Phased administration of gemfibrozil 600 mg bid, then niacin 250 mg/d titrate to 3,000 mg/d, then cholestramine to 16 g/d	13% vs. 26% for hospitalization for angina, MI, TIA, stroke, death, and CV procedures over placebo
Bezafibrate Infarction Prevention	CAD with LDL < 180 and HDL < 45, triglycerides < 300, total cholesterol 180–250	3,090	Benazafibrate vs. placebo	13.6 % vs. 15.0% fatal and nonfatal MI and sudden death ($n = 0.26$) over 6.2 years; but benefits for patients with triglycerides > 200
HATS	CAD with LDL ≤ 145, HDL ≤ 35, and triglycerides < 400	160	Simvastatin 10–20 mg/d + niacin 250 mg bid titrate to 1,000 mg bid	3% vs. 24% (placebo) for CAD death, MI, CVA, or revascularization over 38 months; did not compare combination therapy vs. statin therapy alone
VA-HIT	CAD with LDL ≤ 140 and HDL ≤ 40, and triglyceride ≤ 300	2,531	Gemfibrozil 1,200 mg/d	17% vs. 22% for CAD death and MI over 5.1 years

treatment with fibrates or niacin to reduce the risk of pancreatitis should be initiated before LDL-lowering therapy is recommended.

Patients receiving high-dose statin and fibrate therapy are at higher risk for severe myopathy and hepatocyte injury.

This risk can be minimized by frequent laboratory and symptom monitoring, and the lowering of statin doses.

It is also reasonable to encourage consumption of omega-3 fatty acids in the form of fish oil (dietary modification) or in capsule form (1 g/day) for risk reduction may be reasonable. For treatment of elevated triglycerides, higher doses (2–4 g/day) may be used.

Box 7.4 Therapy of dyslipidemia for secondary prevention

Assess fasting lipid profile in all patients, and within 24 hours of hospitalization for those with an acute cardiovascular or coronary event. For hospitalized patients, initiate lipid-lowering medication as recommended below before d/c according to the following schedule:
- LDL-C should be <100 mg/dl **(I) and** <70 mg/dl is reasonable. **(IIa)**
- If triglycerides are 200–499 mg/dl, non-HDL-C should be <130mg/dl. **(I) and** <100 mg/dl is reasonable. Therapeutic options to reduce non-HDL-C are as follows:
  – more intense LDL-C-lowering therapy; **(I)**
  – niacin or fibrate therapy **after** LDL-C-lowering therapy. **(IIa)**
- If triglycerides are >500 mg/dl, therapeutic options to prevent pancreatitis are fibrate or niacin **before** LDL-lowering therapy; and treat LDL-C to goal **after** triglyceride-lowering therapy. Achieve non-HDL-C <300 mg/dl if possible. **(I)**
  Reasonable to encourage consumption of omega-3 fatty acids for risk reduction. **(IIb)**

Warfarin
A decision to start or continue warfarin in a patient following ACS has to take into consideration the indication, desired intensity of anticoagulation, and concomitant medications. The latter is a particularly important consideration, because antiplatelet therapy (including dual therapy with

aspirin and clopidogrel) has a strong, evidence-based role in secondary prevention, but increases bleeding risks in combination with warfarin.

Atrial fibrillation/flutter

Warfarin should be used to target INR of 2.0–3.0 in post-MI patients with paroxysmal or chronic atrial fibrillation.

Left ventricular mural thrombus

The use of warfarin for known LV thrombus is a class I indication. The ACC/AHA STEMI guidelines recommend at least 3 months of anticoagulation following detection of thrombus, and indefinitely in patients without increased bleeding risk. Our practice is to start warfarin in post-MI patients with an LV thrombus, perform echocardiography in 3–6 months, and consider discontinuation of warfarin in a very select group of patients: those with complete resolution of the thrombus and recovery of LV systolic function to normal or only slightly depressed levels.

Severe left ventricular systolic dysfunction without known thrombus

Retrospective analysis of the SAVE and SOLVD studies along with a corresponding meta-analysis suggests that anticoagulation decreases mortality and stroke risk in post-MI patients with LV systolic dysfunction. A decreased in LVEF of 5% was associated with an 18% relative increase in stroke risk, and anticoagulation was associated with a lower stroke risk in the SAVE trial. However, retrospective analysis of the VHeFT II study did not suggest anticoagulation reduces in events in patients with HF. Furthermore, the rate of LV thrombus after large anterior AMI appears to be decreasing with increasing use of reperfusion therapy and ACE inhibitors; one study found the prevalence of thrombi of 13 out of a cohort of 309 patients within 2 weeks by echocardiogram.[20]

Overall, the evidence for anticoagulation for severe LV dysfunction is limited; a Cochrane review cautions that currently there is only data available from one pilot RCT and preliminary results from one large RCT to indicate suggest that oral anticoagulation is beneficial. Until the results of RCTs are reported, the decision to anticoagulate for severe LV systolic dysfunction/severe regional wall motion abnormalities requires clinical judgment in lieu of established evidence. The STEMI guidelines state that it is reasonable (class IIa) to prescribe warfarin to post-STEMI patients with LV dysfunction and extensive regional wall motion abnormalities; it is a class IIb indication to consider warfarin in patients with severe LV dysfunction alone, with or without CHF.

A reasonable approach in a post-MI patient with apical LV hypokinesis/akinesis or extensive anterior akinesis is to prescribe warfarin, adjusted to an INR 2.0–3.0 for 6 months. Repeat echocardiography can then be performed, and unless an LV thrombus or worsening LV systolic function is seen at that time, warfarin can be discontinued.

Anticoagulation with and without antiplatelet therapy after AMI

The APRICOT II trial found that patients <75 years old with STEMI treated with fibrinolytics treated with moderate-intensity warfarin (INR 2.0–3.0) and aspirin 80 mg had a 20% absolute risk, 23% relative risk reduction for the combined endpoint of death, MI, and revascularization compared with aspirin 80 mg alone at 3 months.[21]

The WARIS II study found that patients <75 years old with STEMI treated with high-intensity warfarin (INR 2.8–4.2) had a 5% absolute risk, 19% relative risk reduction for a combined endpoint of death, MI, and stroke, and that moderate-intensity warfarin (INR 2.022.5) plus aspirin 75 mg had a 3.3% absolute risk, 29% relative risk reduction for the combined endpoint compared with aspirin 160 mg alone, but at a higher risk of bleeding.[22]

The ASPECT II study found that for patients with MI or USA within 8 weeks treated with high-intensity warfarin (INR 3–4) had a lower risk of combined endpoint of death, MI, or stroke (5% absolute), and moderate-intensity warfarin (INR 2.0–2.5) plus aspirin 80 mg also had a lower risk of combined endpoints (5% absolute) compared with aspirin 80 mg alone. Both warfarin and warfarin–aspirin therapy had a higher risk of minor bleeding.[23]

Two trials (CARS and LoWASA) did not find a benefit associated with combination low-dose (INR < 2) warfarin and aspirin therapy for reducing death, MI, or stroke.[24,25]

The ACC/AHA STEMI guidelines suggest a detailed approach for combination anticoagulation-antiplatelet therapy (Figure 7.3).

Influenza vaccination

In 2006, the AHA/ACC recommended annual influenza vaccination in patients with coronary vascular disease, for the secondary prevention of CV events. The FLUVACS study randomized 201 patients hospitalized for MI or PCI to influenza vaccination or no vaccination. There was a significant reduction in CV death (2% vs. 8%) and the composite endpoint of CV death, MI, or ischemia (11% vs. 23%) at 1 year.[26]

Medications of limited benefit to patients following ACS

Vitamins/antioxidants

Antioxidant vitamins supplementation has been studied extensively in multiple randomized clinical trials (e.g., the HOPE study and the Heart Protection Study); no clear benefit has been observed for vitamin supplementation therapy to reduce future CV events. Therefore, the current guidelines state that antioxidant vitamins such as vitamin E and/or vitamin C should not be prescribed.

The NORVIT trial randomized 3,749 patients after MI to combinations of folic acid, vitamin B6, and vitamin B12 versus placebo. While mean total homocysteine levels were decreased with folic acid and B12, no benefits were observed on the primary endpoints of MI, stroke, and sudden death; in fact, treatment with all three vitamins was associated with higher risk. In a study of folate, vitamin B6, and vitamin B12 after coronary stent placement, there was increased risk of in-stent restenosis and target-vessel revascularization.[27]

Estrogen replacement therapy

The HERS trial and HERS II follow-up demonstrated that hormone replacement therapy (HRT) with estrogen and

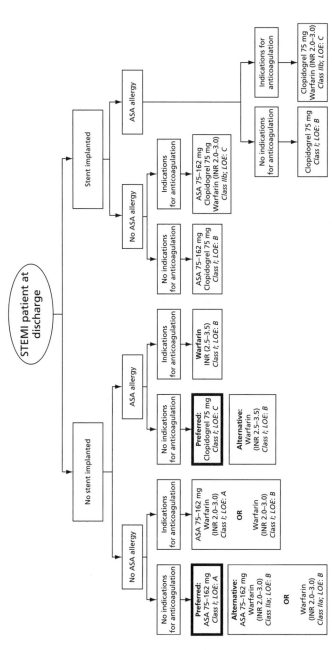

Figure 7.3 ACC/AHA guidelines for use the antiplatelet and anticoagulation therapy after STEMI (adapted, with permission, from Antman et al. *J Am Coll Cardiol* 2004; 44: E1–E211[53]).

progestin compared with placebo in postmenopausal women did not reduce risk for coronary death or nonfatal MI over an average of 4.1 years of follow-up.[28] However, an increase in the incidence of venous thromboembolism and gall bladder disease was seen.

The Women's Health Initiative (WHI) supported two trials. The first study considered estrogen and progestin in post-menopausal women with an intact uterus, and found that estrogen/progestin may have increased the risk of coronary events, especially during the first year after beginning hormone therapy.[29] Another study, which considered estrogen alone in women following a hysterectomy, was stopped early because of increased strokes in the hormone replacement arm, and found no decreased risk of coronary events.[30] Based on these data, the current guidelines recommend the following:

- Starting estrogen with progestin for cardioprotective benefits in women after myocardial infarction.
- Stopping estrogen with progestin in woman on that therapy at the time of a myocardial infarction.

The guidelines note that if a woman has been on HRT for over 1–2 years and wishes to continue this therapy for another compelling indication, she should be counseled on a higher risk of cardiovascular events. In such patients, HRT is *strongly discouraged* during bed rest in the hospital, because of an increased risk of venous thromboembolism.

Nonsteroidal anti-inflammatory agents and related compounds

Nonsteroidal anti-inflammatory drugs (NSAIDs) are thought to inhibit the actions of aspirin, which has consequences for post-MI patients prescribed aspirin for secondary prevention. No RCTs examining the use of NSAIDs and aspirin are available, and observational studies are inconsistent. Data from the Physicians Health Study suggest that among patients who randomized to aspirin, the use of an NSAID for more than 60 days per year increased the risk for a first MI.

Much controversy surrounds the COX-2 inhibitors and risk for cardiovascular events. Rofecoxib (Vioxx) was withdrawn for use in 2004. Data from the APPROVe trial to prevent adenomatous colonic polyps and meta-analyses of smaller trials consistently suggest increased risk for MI and stroke associated with rofexocib therapy. Data from the Adenoma Prevention with Celexocib (APC) trial and the Prevention of Spontaneous Adenomatous Polyps (PreSAP) trials suggest that cardiovascular death, MI, stroke, or HF was highest in the group taking 400 mg bid and lowest in the group taking 400 mg daily compared with placebo.[32] Of note, the APC trial was discontinued early by its data-safety monitoring board for the increase in cardiovascular risk. The increased risk due to celexocib was seen particularly in patients with preexisting coronary artery disease.

A statement by the AHA suggested that in patients with or at high risk for cardiovascular disease, COX-2 inhibitors should "be limited to patients for whom there are no appropriate alternatives; and then only in the lowest dose and for the shortest duration necessary." The ACC/AHA STEMI guidelines recommend discontinuing the use of NSAIDs or Cox-2 inhibitors in patients who are having STEMI.

Nonpharmacologic measures

Antiarrhythmic devices

General considerations
Patients with prior MI resulting in ischemic cardiomyopathy and heart failure are at high risk for sudden death from ventricular tachyarryrthmias. Selected patients after ACS (in particular, those with large STEMI) may benefit from having an implantable cardioverter defibrillator (ICD) placed, with specific criteria based on data from several RCTs (Table 7.9). The detailed review of this topic is beyond the scope of this handbook, and the readers are referred to the AHA/ACC/ESC 2006 Guidelines for Management of Patients With Ventricular Arrhythmias and the Prevention of Sudden Cardiac Death. The brief summary is provided below.[33]

Table 7.9 Major RCTs of ICD therapy after MI

Study	Population	n	Dose/titration	Effectiveness
MUSTT	MI, LVEF ≤ 40%, NSVT, inducible VT/VF on EPS	704	Primary: EPS guided antiarrhythmic therapy vs. none	25% vs. 32% of cardiac arrest or death over 5 years
MADIT	MI, LVEF ≤ 35%, NSVT, inducible VT/VF on EPS	196	ICD vs. medical therapy	27 months
MADIT II	MI, LVEF ≤ 30%	1,232	ICD vs. medical therapy	14.2% vs. 19.8% for all-cause death over 20 months
DINAMIT	MI within 6–40 days, LVEF ≤ 35%, and reduced HR variability or HR ≥ 80	674	ICD vs. none	No significant difference 6.9% vs. 7.5% for annual all-cause mortality over 30 months
SCD-HeFT	Ischemic or nonischemic cardiomyopathy, LVEF ≤ 35%, NYHA II–III	2,521	ICD vs. placebo	22% vs. 29% for all-cause death over 46 months

The initial MADIT study (MADIT I) found that post-MI patients with LVEF ≤ 35% and inducible VT on electrophysiologic study (EPS) had improved survival with ICD implantation, compared with conventional medical therapy.[34] The MUSTT study of post-MI patients with LVEF < 40% randomized patients to EPS-guided therapy or standard medical therapy. Here, EPS-guided therapy consisted of either antiarrhythmic medications shown to suppress ventricular tachyarrhythmias during EPS, or ICD implantation. Patients assigned to EPS-guided therapy had lower rates of SCD.[35] Importantly, the mortality benefit was limited to patient who received ICDs. The MADIT II study considered post-MI patients with LVEF 30%, a population presumably at high risk for SCD and deemed not to need EPS for further risk stratification. This study demonstrated that these patients derived a survival advantage from an ICD, although this may have been a lower-risk population compared with MUSTT and the MADIT I populations.[36]

The SCD-HeFT trial also did not require inducible VT on EPS, but was restricted to patients with symptomatic heart failure (NYHA class II–III) of either ischemic or nonischemic etiology. ICD implantation was associated with a significant decrease in all-cause mortality compared with medical therapy.[37]

Box 7.5 Cardiac resynchronization therapy (CRT)

Class I
- For patients who have LV ejection fraction (LVEF) less than or equal to 35%, a QRS duration greater than or equal to 0.12 seconds, and sinus rhythm, CRT with or without an ICD is indicated for the treatment of New York Heart Association (NYHA) functional Class III or ambulatory Class IV heart failure symptoms with optimal recommended medical therapy.

Class IIa
- For patients who have LVEF less than or equal to 35%, a QRS duration greater than or equal to 0.12 seconds, and atrial fibrillation of , CRT with or without ICT is reasonable for the treatment of NYHA functional Class III or ambulatory Class IV heart failure symptoms on optimal recommended medical therapy.
- For patients with LVEF less than or equal to 35% with NYHA functional Class III or ambulatory Class IV symptoms who are receiving optimal recommended medical therapy and who have frequent dependence on ventricular pacing, CRT is reasonable.

Class IIb
- For patients with LVEF less than or equal to 35% with NYHA functional Class I or II symptoms who are receiving optimal recommended medical therapy, undergoing implantation of a permanent pacemaker and/or ICD, with anticipated frequent ventricular pacing, CRT may be considered.

Timing of ICD implantation

The DINAMIT study examined ICD implantation in patients with LVEF ≤ 35% within 40 days of acute MI, but failed to demonstrate a significant benefit for ICD within this time period.[38] The CABG-PATCH trial found no evidence of improved survival for patients with CAD, LVEF ≤ 36%, and an abnormal signal-averaged electrocardiogram, in whom an ICD was placed at time of elective CABG.[39] Based on these studies, the clinical practice is to withhold placement of ICD *for primary prevention* of SCD until at least 40 days after a myocardial infarction, and 3 months after last coronary revascularization (CABG or PCI).

Therapy of comorbidities following ACS

Diabetes mellitus

As discussed in Chapter 5, diabetes confers a significant additional risk of mortality during ACS. Following hospital discharge of a diabetic patient with ACS, meticulous control of serum glucose becomes paramount. The overall goal is to control blood glucose to goal HbA1c < 7%. A combination of diet, physical activity prescription, oral hypoglycemic agents, and insulin may be use.

Ten-year follow-up from the United Kingdom Prospective Diabetes Study (UKPDS) of Type II diabetics demonstrated a continued reduction in microvascular risk and emergent risk reductions for myocardial infarction and death from any cause. Data from the ACCORD has added uncertainty to optimal blood glucose targets. The trial randomized type 2 diabetics to targets of HbA1c < 6% versus 7–9%. The trial was stopped early due to higher deaths in the intensive treatment group compared with standard therapy; of note, there were fewer nonfatal MIs in the intenstive treatment group even though there were more deaths in total.[40] The most recent ADVANCE trial did not find an increased risk with intensive glucose lowering, but again failed to demonstrate a statistically significant benefit.[41]

An important consideration for diabetic patients is that thiazolinediones ("glitazones") may cause substantial sodium and fluid retention, and thus are generally contraindicated in patients with decompensated (NYHA Class III–IV) congestive heart failure after ACS.

Box 7.6 Secondary prevention guidelines

- Initiate lifestyle and pharmacotherapy to achieve near-normal HbA1c.
- Begin vigorous modification of other risk factors: physical activity;
  - weight management;
  - blood pressure control;
  - cholesterol management.
- Coordinate diabetic care with patient's primary care physician or endocrinologist.

Hypertension

Guidelines from both the AHA/ACC and the JNC 7 recommend blood pressure targets of <140/90 in general, and <130/80 in particular for patients with hypertension and diabetes or renal disease. The 2003 European Society of Hypertension – European Society of Cardiology guidelines recommend a BP goal of 130/85 in high-risk patients with CAD. Many of the previously discussed data-driven pharmacologic regimens for secondary prevention of ACS reduce blood pressure as well (beta-blockers, ACE inhibitors, ARBs, and aldosterone antagonists). If target blood pressure is still not achieved after institution of this regimen, the addition of thiazide diuretic and/or a dihydropiridine-type calcium channel blocker should be considered. An investigation of the possible cause of secondary hypertension, particularly primary hyperaldosteronism, renal artery stenosis, and pheochromocytoma, should be strongly considered in any patient with resistant or accelerated hypertension.

Depression

Major depression is common among patients hospitalized for CAD (incidence 17–27%).[42] Depression after MI is associated with a 5.7-fold increase in cardiac mortality within 6 months.[43]

The ENRICHD study found that a combination of short-term individual cognitive behavior therapy and sertraline, when needed, reduced depressive symptoms over 6 months in depressed or socially isolated patients after MI.[44] The CREATE trial found that citalopram was superior to placebo in reducing depressive symptoms, while finding no evidence of a benefit of interpersonal psychotherapy over clinical management.[45]

Citalopram or sertraline plus clinical management could be considered as a first-step treatment for patients with CAD and major depression. However, neither the ENRICHD or CREATE trials found that SSRIs reduced mortality or recurrent MI, and additional research on clinical outcomes is needed.

Lifestyle recommendations following ACS

General physical activity and structured cardiac rehabilitation

After acute coronary syndrome, most patients will benefit from structured, medically supervised cardiac rehabilitation programs. In general, these programs consist of exercise-based therapy, but may include also risk factor reduction (i.e., smoking cessation and stress reduction) and psychological support. The benefits of exercise after MI are not completely understood and are likely multifactorial with to respect effects on the coronary vasculature, autonomic tome, and inflammatory markers, as well as effects on risk-factor profiles.

A meta-analysis of exercise programs reports a typical regiment of several hour-long sessions per week of graded exercise at approximately 75% of maximum intensity over a period of months to years.[46] Patients in exercise programs had lower risk for all-cause and cardiac mortality, and improved risk-factor profiles (lipids, blood pressure, smoking cessation) compared with patients receiving usual care.

Box 7.7 Physical activity after ACS

Assess risk with an activity history and/or an exercise test, to guide exercise prescription:

- **aerobic activity goal:** 30–60 minutes of moderate-intensity activity (brisk walking) $\geq$5 days per week;
- **resistance training goals:** 2 days per week.

Advise medically supervised programs for high-risk patients (e.g., recent acute coronary syndrome or revascularization, heart failure).

Sexual activity after ACS

Recommendations for resuming sexual intercourse after ACS have been proposed by the 2005 Second Princeton Consensus Panel.[47] Patients who have undergone successful revascularization and without exercise-induced ischemia can probably resume sexual activity within 3–4 weeks post MI. Unrevascularized patients without exercise-induced ischemia can probably resume sexual activity within 6–8 weeks. Unrevascularized patients with MI within 2–6 weeks are at intermediate risk and can evaluated with stress testing. Patients with MI within 2 weeks are at high risk and should be risk-stratified before restarting sexual activity.

Phosphodiesterase-5 inhibitors (sildenafil, vardenafil, tadalafil) are used for erectile dysfunction, but are contraindicated with the concurrent use of nitrates. Patients should not use nitrates within 24 hours of sildenafil or vardenafil, or within 48 hours of tadalafil.

Smoking cessation

Smoking increases the incidence of coronary spasm and ischemic episodes in patients with CAD.[48] All patients with MI should have their smoking history assessed and be advised to cease smoking. Patients should also attempt to reduce their exposure to secondhand smoke.

Box 7.8 Smoking cessation after ACS

- Ask about tobacco use status at every visit.
- Advise every tobacco user to quit.
- Assess the tobacco user's willingness to quit.
- Assist by counseling and developing a plan for quitting.
- Arrange follow-up, referral to special programs, or pharmacotherapy, including nicotine replacement, varenicline, and bupropion.
- Urge avoidance of exposure to environmental tobacco smoke at work and home.

Diet/nutrition and weight loss

The AHA has published general recommendations for reducing cardiovascular disease risk (see below). In addition, patients with diabetes mellitus should consider ADA diet recommendations, and patients with hypertension should consider JNC 7 DASH diet recommendations.

The **metabolic syndrome** (see Chapter 5) has been associated with increased risk for cardiovascular disease and type 2 diabetes mellitus. Patients with metabolic syndrome hospitalized for myocardial infarction have higher incidence of in-hospital death and severe heart failure.[49] While no particular therapies are suggested for secondary prevention after ACS for metabolic syndrome patients, the prior study suggested that hyperglycemia was correlated with the development of heart failure. The AHA recommends smoking cessation, and control of lipids, blood pressure, and glucose levels to the recommended levels, as well as weight loss to achieve a BMI less than 25 kg/m^2 and increased physical activity.

Box 7.9 General diet and weight loss recommendations after ACS

Diet
- Start dietary therapy. Reduce intake of saturated fats (to ≤7% of total calories) *trans*-fatty acids, and cholesterol (to <20 mg/d).

- Adding plant stanols/sterols (2 g/d) and viscous fiber (≥10 g/d) will further lower LDL-C.
- Encourage increased consumption of omega-3 fatty acids in the form of fish or in capsule form (1 g/d) for risk reduction.
- Minimize intake of beverages and foods with added sugars.
- Choose and prepare foods with little or no salt.

Weight loss
- Assess body mass index (BMI) and waist circumference on each visit and consistently encourage weight maintenance/reduction through an appropriate balance of physical activity, calorie intake, and behavioral programs to maintain/achieve a body mass index between 18.5 and 24.9 kg/m². **(I)**
- If waist circumference (at the iliac crest) is 35 inches in women and 40 inches in men, initiate lifestyle changes and consider treatment strategies for metabolic syndrome as indicated. **(I)**
- The initial goal of weight loss therapy should be to reduce body weight by approximately 10% from baseline. With success, further weight loss can be attempted if indicated through further assessment. **(I)**

Alcohol
Dietary studies have consistently demonstrated a J-shaped relationship between the amount of routinely consumed alcohol and cardiovascular events, including ACS and stroke. Moderate consumption (0.5–1.0 drinks daily for women, 1–2 drinks daily for men) increases HDL levels and has positive effects on post-prandial glucose and insulin levels. Moderate consumption of ethanol has been associated with reduced risk of recurrent events after MI. However, the AHA reinforces that "unlike other potentially beneficial dietary components, the consumption of alcohol cannot be recommended solely for CVD risk reduction," and recommends that "if alcoholic beverages are consumed, they should be limited to no more than 2 drinks per day for

men and 1 drink per day for women, and ideally should be consumed with meals."[50]

Fish oil

The relationship between fish consumption, fish oil, and omega-3 fatty acids continues to be under investigation. Evidence from prospective secondary prevention studies suggests that EPA+DHA supplementation either as fatty fish or supplements reduces subsequent cardiac and all-cause mortality.[51] However, the results of a systematic review found the existing data were too limited to provide reliable effect size estimates for dietary changes, including fish oil consumption.[52]

AHA recommendations in 2006 are that patients with documented CHD are advised to consume approximately 1 g of EPA-DHA per day, preferably from oily fish, although EPA-DHA supplements could be considered in consultation with their physician. For individuals with hypertrigly-ceridemia, 2–4 g of EPA-DHA per day, provided as capsules under a physician's care, are recommended.

References

1. Jokhadar M, Jacobsen SJ, Reeder GS, Weston SA, Roger VL. Sudden death and recurrent ischemic events after myocardial infarction in the community. *Am J Epidemiol* 2004; 159: 1040–6.
2. A randomised, blinded, trial of clopidogrel versus aspirin in patients at risk of ischaemic events (CAPRIE). CAPRIE Steering Committee. *Lancet* 1996; 348: 1329–39.
3. Yusuf S, Zhao F, Mehta SR, Chrolavicius S, Tognoni G, Fox KK. Effects of clopidogrel in addition to aspirin in patients with acute coronary syndromes without ST-segment elevation. *N Engl J Med* 2001; 345: 494–502.
4. Mehta SR, Yusuf S, Peters RJ, *et al*. Effects of pretreatment with clopidogrel and aspirin followed by long-term therapy in patients undergoing percutaneous coronary intervention: the PCI-CURE study. *Lancet* 2001; 358: 527–33.
5. Steinhubl SR, Berger PB, Mann JT, 3rd, *et al*. Early and sustained dual oral antiplatelet therapy following percutaneous coronary intervention: a randomized controlled trial. *Jama* 2002; 288: 2411–20.
6. Bhatt DL, Fox KA, Hacke W, *et al*. Clopidogrel and aspirin versus aspirin alone for the prevention of atherothrombotic events. *N Engl J Med* 2006; 354: 1706–17.

7. Freemantle N, Cleland J, Young P, Mason J, Harrison J. Beta blockade after myocardial infarction: systematic review and meta regression analysis. *Bmj* 1999; 318: 1730–7.

8. Tognoni G, Franzosi MG. AIRE Extension (AIREX) study. *Lancet* 1997; 350: 366–7.

9. Braunwald E, Domanski MJ, Fowler SE, et al. Angiotensin-converting-enzyme inhibition in stable coronary artery disease. *N Engl J Med* 2004; 351: 2058–68.

10. Pfeffer MA, McMurray JJ, Velazquez EJ, et al. Valsartan, captopril, or both in myocardial infarction complicated by heart failure, left ventricular dysfunction, or both. *N Engl J Med* 2003; 349: 1893–906.

11. Pitt B, Poole-Wilson PA, Segal R, et al. Effect of losartan compared with captopril on mortality in patients with symptomatic heart failure: randomised trial—the Losartan Heart Failure Survival Study ELITE II. *Lancet* 2000; 355: 1582–7.

12. Granger CB, McMurray JJ, Yusuf S, et al. Effects of candesartan in patients with chronic heart failure and reduced left-ventricular systolic function intolerant to angiotensin-converting-enzyme inhibitors: the CHARM-Alternative trial. *Lancet* 2003; 362: 772–6.

13. Dickstein K, Kjekshus J. Effects of losartan and captopril on mortality and morbidity in high-risk patients after acute myocardial infarction: the OPTIMAAL randomised trial. Optimal Trial in Myocardial Infarction with Angiotensin II Antagonist Losartan. *Lancet* 2002; 360: 752–60.

14. McMurray JJ, Ostergren J, Swedberg K, et al. Effects of candesartan in patients with chronic heart failure and reduced left-ventricular systolic function taking angiotensin-converting-enzyme inhibitors: the CHARM-Added trial. *Lancet* 2003; 362: 767–71.

15. Pitt B, Remme W, Zannad F, et al. Eplerenone, a selective aldosterone blocker, in patients with left ventricular dysfunction after myocardial infarction. *N Engl J Med* 2003; 348: 1309–21.

16. Cannon CP, Braunwald E, McCabe CH, et al. Intensive versus moderate lipid lowering with statins after acute coronary syndromes. *N Engl J Med* 2004; 350: 1495–504.

17. Schwartz GG, Olsson AG, Ezekowitz MD, et al. Effects of atorvastatin on early recurrent ischemic events in acute coronary syndromes: the MIRACL study: a randomized controlled trial. *Jama* 2001; 285: 1711–8.

18. Canner PL, Berge KG, Wenger NK, et al. Fifteen year mortality in Coronary Drug Project patients: long-term benefit with niacin. *J Am Coll Cardiol* 1986; 8: 1245–55.

19. Rubins HB, Robins SJ, Collins D, et al. Gemfibrozil for the secondary prevention of coronary heart disease in men with low levels of high-density lipoprotein cholesterol. Veterans Affairs

High-Density Lipoprotein Cholesterol Intervention Trial Study Group. *N Engl J Med* 1999; 341: 410–8.

20. Greaves SC, Zhi G, Lee RT, *et al*. Incidence and natural history of left ventricular thrombus following anterior wall acute myocardial infarction. *Am J Cardiol* 1997; 80: 442–8.

21. Brouwer MA, van den Bergh PJ, Aengevaeren WR, *et al*. Aspirin plus coumarin versus aspirin alone in the prevention of reocclusion after fibrinolysis for acute myocardial infarction: results of the Antithrombotics in the Prevention of Reocclusion In Coronary Thrombolysis (APRICOT)-2 Trial. *Circulation* 2002; 106: 659–65.

22. Hurlen M, Abdelnoor M, Smith P, Erikssen J, Arnesen H. Warfarin, aspirin, or both after myocardial infarction. *N Engl J Med* 2002; 347: 969–74.

23. van Es RF, Jonker JJ, Verheugt FW, Deckers JW, Grobbee DE. Aspirin and coumadin after acute coronary syndromes (the ASPECT-2 study): a randomised controlled trial. *Lancet* 2002; 360: 109–13.

24. Randomised double-blind trial of fixed low-dose warfarin with aspirin after myocardial infarction. Coumadin Aspirin Reinfarction Study (CARS) Investigators. *Lancet* 1997; 350: 389–96.

25. Herlitz J, Holm J, Peterson M, Karlson BW, Haglid Evander M, Erhardt L. Effect of fixed low-dose warfarin added to aspirin in the long term after acute myocardial infarction; the LoWASA Study. *Eur Heart J* 2004; 25: 232–9.

26. Gurfinkel EP, de la Fuente RL, Mendiz O, Mautner B. Influenza vaccine pilot study in acute coronary syndromes and planned percutaneous coronary interventions: the FLU Vaccination Acute Coronary Syndromes (FLUVACS) Study. *Circulation* 2002; 105: 2143–7.

27. Bonaa KH, Njolstad I, Ueland PM, *et al*. Homocysteine lowering and cardiovascular events after acute myocardial infarction. *N Engl J Med* 2006; 354: 1578–88.

28. Grady D, Herrington D, Bittner V, *et al*. Cardiovascular disease outcomes during 6.8 years of hormone therapy: Heart and Estrogen/progestin Replacement Study follow-up (HERS II). *Jama* 2002; 288: 49–57.

29. Wassertheil-Smoller S, Hendrix SL, Limacher M, *et al*. Effect of estrogen plus progestin on stroke in postmenopausal women: the Women's Health Initiative: a randomized trial. *Jama* 2003; 289: 2673–84.

30. Anderson GL, Limacher M, Assaf AR, *et al*. Effects of conjugated equine estrogen in postmenopausal women with hysterectomy: the Women's Health Initiative randomized controlled trial. *Jama* 2004; 291: 1701–12.

31. Bresalier RS, Sandler RS, Quan H, *et al*. Cardiovascular events associated with rofecoxib in a colorectal adenoma chemoprevention trial. *N Engl J Med* 2005; 352: 1092–102.

32. Solomon SD, Pfeffer MA, McMurray JJ, *et al*. Effect of celecoxib on cardiovascular events and blood pressure in two trials for the prevention of colorectal adenomas. *Circulation* 2006; 114: 1028–35.

33. Zipes DP, Camm AJ, Borggrefe M, *et al*. ACC/AHA/ESC 2006 Guidelines for Management of Patients With Ventricular Arrhythmias and the Prevention of Sudden Cardiac Death: a report of the American College of Cardiology/American Heart Association Task Force and the European Society of Cardiology Committee for Practice Guidelines (writing committee to develop Guidelines for Management of Patients With Ventricular Arrhythmias and the Prevention of Sudden Cardiac Death): developed in collaboration with the European Heart Rhythm Association and the Heart Rhythm Society. *Circulation* 2006; 114: e385–e484.

34. Moss AJ, Hall WJ, Cannom DS, *et al*. Improved survival with an implanted defibrillator in patients with coronary disease at high risk for ventricular arrhythmia. Multicenter Automatic Defibrillator Implantation Trial Investigators. *N Engl J Med* 1996; 335: 1933–40.

35. Buxton AE, Lee KL, Fisher JD, Josephson ME, Prystowsky EN, Hafley G. A randomized study of the prevention of sudden death in patients with coronary artery disease. Multicenter Unsustained Tachycardia Trial Investigators. *N Engl J Med* 1999; 341: 1882–90.

36. Moss AJ, Zareba W, Hall WJ, *et al*. Prophylactic implantation of a defibrillator in patients with myocardial infarction and reduced ejection fraction. *N Engl J Med* 2002; 346: 877–83.

37. Bardy GH, Lee KL, Mark DB, *et al*. Amiodarone or an implantable cardioverter–defibrillator for congestive heart failure. *N Engl J Med* 2005; 352: 225–37.

38. Hohnloser SH, Kuck KH, Dorian P, *et al*. Prophylactic use of an implantable cardioverter–defibrillator after acute myocardial infarction. *N Engl J Med* 2004; 351: 2481–8.

39. Bigger JT, Jr. Prophylactic use of implanted cardiac defibrillators in patients at high risk for ventricular arrhythmias after coronary-artery bypass graft surgery. Coronary Artery Bypass Graft (CABG) Patch Trial Investigators. *N Engl J Med* 1997; 337: 1569–75.

40. Gerstein HC, Riddle MC, Kendall DM, *et al*. Glycemia treatment strategies in the Action to Control Cardiovascular Risk in Diabetes (ACCORD) trial. *Am J Cardiol* 2007; 99: 34i–43i.

41. Patel A, MacMahon S, Chalmers J, *et al*. Intensive blood glucose control and vascular outcomes in patients with type 2 diabetes. *N Engl J Med* 2008; 358: 2560–72.

42. Rudisch B, Nemeroff CB. Epidemiology of comorbid coronary artery disease and depression. *Biol Psychiatry* 2003; 54: 227–40.

43. Frasure-Smith N, Lesperance F, Talajic M. Depression following myocardial infarction. Impact on 6-month survival. *Jama* 1993; 270: 1819–25.
44. Berkman LF, Blumenthal J, Burg M, *et al*. Effects of treating depression and low perceived social support on clinical events after myocardial infarction: the Enhancing Recovery in Coronary Heart Disease Patients (ENRICHD) Randomized Trial. *Jama* 2003; 289: 3106–16.
45. Lesperance F, Frasure-Smith N, Koszycki D, *et al*. Effects of citalopram and interpersonal psychotherapy on depression in patients with coronary artery disease: the Canadian Cardiac Randomized Evaluation of Antidepressant and Psychotherapy Efficacy (CREATE) trial. *Jama* 2007; 297: 367–79.
46. Taylor RS, Brown A, Ebrahim S, *et al*. Exercise-based rehabilitation for patients with coronary heart disease: systematic review and meta-analysis of randomized controlled trials. *Am J Med* 2004; 116: 682–92.
47. Kostis JB, Jackson G, Rosen R, *et al*. Sexual dysfunction and cardiac risk (the Second Princeton Consensus Conference). *Am J Cardiol* 2005; 96: 85M–93M.
48. Barry J, Mead K, Nabel EG, *et al*. Effect of smoking on the activity of ischemic heart disease. *Jama* 1989; 261: 398–402.
49. Zeller M, Steg PG, Ravisy J, *et al*. Prevalence and impact of metabolic syndrome on hospital outcomes in acute myocardial infarction. *Arch Intern Med* 2005; 165: 1192–8.
50. Goldberg IJ, Mosca L, Piano MR, Fisher EA. AHA Science Advisory: Wine and your heart: a science advisory for healthcare professionals from the Nutrition Committee, Council on Epidemiology and Prevention, and Council on Cardiovascular Nursing of the American Heart Association. *Circulation* 2001; 103: 472–5.
51. Kris-Etherton PM, Harris WS, Appel LJ. Fish consumption, fish oil, omega-3 fatty acids, and cardiovascular disease. *Circulation* 2002; 106: 2747–57.
52. Iestra JA, Kromhout D, van der Schouw YT, Grobbee DE, Boshuizen HC, van Staveren WA. Effect size estimates of lifestyle and dietary changes on all-cause mortality in coronary artery disease patients: a systematic review. *Circulation* 2005; 112: 924–34.
53. Antman EM, Anbe DT, Armstrong PW, *et al*. ACC/AHA guidelines for the management of patients with ST-elevation myocardial infarction; A report of the American College of Cardiology/ American Heart Association Task Force on Practice Guidelines (Committee to Revise the 1999 Guidelines for the Management of Patients with Acute Myocardial Infarction). *J Am Coll Cardiol* 2004; 44: E1–E211.

Appendix

(Figures A.1–A.7 adapted from Wellens HJJ and Conover M, *The ECG in Emergency Decision Making (second edition)*. Copyright © 2006, Elsevier Inc.)

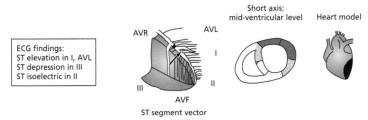

Figure A.1 ECG in anterior wall MI: LAD occlusion between the first septal perforator and the first diagonal branch results in anterolateral ischemia, but the basal anterior septum is preserved. The ST-segment deviation vector points to the dominant ischemic area.

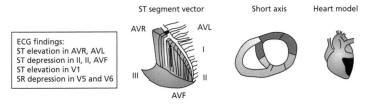

Figure A.2 ECG in anterior wall MI: LAD occlusion proximal to the first septal and diagonal branches results in a large anteroseptal and anterolateral ischemia. The ST-segment deviation vector points at the base of the heart.

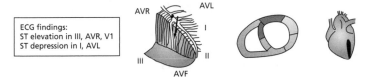

Figure A.3 ECG in anterior wall MI: LAD occlusion distal to the first diagonal branch but proximal to the first septal branch results in dominant anteroseptal ischemia, with the ST-segment deviation vector pointing inferior and to the right.

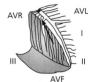

ECG findings:
ST elevation in AVR > St elevation in V1
ST depression in II, II, and AVF
ST depressions in precordial leads to the left of V_2

Figure A.4 ECG in the left main coronary artery: occlusion results in global LV ischemia in both LAD and LCx distributions. The ST-segment deviation vector points at the base of the heart. ST depressions in the precordial leads to the left of V_2 represent posterior wall ischemia, mostly seen in V_4.

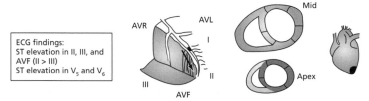

ECG findings:
ST elevation in II, III, and AVF (II > III)
ST elevation in V_5 and V_6

Figure A.5 ECG in anterior wall MI: distal LAD occlusion results in inferopaical ischemia. The ST-segment deviation vector points inferiorly and to the left.

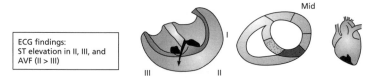

ECG findings:
ST elevation in II, III, and AVF (II > III)

Figure A.6 ECG in inferior wall MI: RCA occlusion results in inferior or inferoposterior ischemia. The ST-segment deviation vector points inferiorly and to lead III, resulting in ST elevation in III > II. With a proximal RCA occlusion, ST-segment elevation in leads V_1 and V_4R with positive T waves indicates RV involvement. When ischemia extends posteriorly, ST depressions are seen in the precordial elads. With a distal RCA occlusion, the ST segment in V_4R is isoelectric, with a positive T wave.

ECG findings:
ST elevation in II, III, and
AVF (II > III)
ST elevation in V_5 and V_6

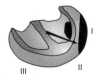

Figure A.7 ECG in inferior wall MI: LCx occlusion results in inferolateral ischemia. The ST-segment deviation vector points inferiorly and to lead II, resulting in ST elevation in II > III. When ischemia extends to the lateral wall, ST elevations are seen in I, AVL, V_5, and V_6. With posterior wall extension, ST depressions are seen in precordial leads.

Proposed rapid desensitization protocol #1 (duration 3.5 hours)

1 Admit to CCU. Monitor BP, HR, Peak Exp Flow q30 minutes. Have benadryl, solumedrol, epinephrine available.
2 Administer 1 mg aspirin. Monitor.
3 Double dose every 30 minutes (total of eight doses).
4 Final dose 100 mg.
5 Observed in CCU 3 hours after the last dose for development of late allergic reaction.

Proposed rapid desensitization protocol #2 (duration 2.5 hours)

1 Admit to CCU. Monitor BP, HR, Peak Exp Flow q30 minutes. Have benadryl, solumedrol, epinephrine available.
2 Administer 5 mg aspirin. Monitor.
3 Double dose every 30 minutes (total of five doses).
4 Final dose 75 mg.
5 Observed in CCU 3 hours after the last dose for development of late allergic reaction.

Figure A.8 F Aspirin desensitization protocol (from Silberman et al. AJC 2005; 95(4): 509–10). Immediate tolerance on 88% of patients. If an allergic reaction develops, it is successfully treated, and patients can be rechallenged after 48 hours. Should aspirin use be interrupted after PCI (stopped for elective surgery), repeat desensitization may be needed.

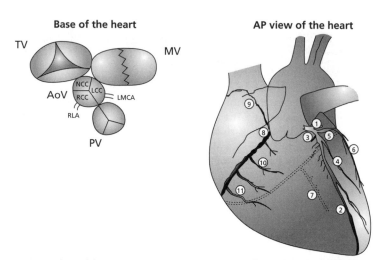

Figure A.9 Coronary anatomy: a schematic of the base of the heart and the relationships between than tricuspid valve (TV), the mitral valve (MV), the aortic valve (AoV), and the pulmonic valve (PV), as well as the origins of the left main coronary artery (LMCA) from the left coronary cusp of the partic valve (LCC) and of the right coronary artery (RCA) from the right coronary cusp of the aortic valve (RCC), are shown. NCC is the noncoronary cusp. The locations of the major coronary arteries are shown in a schematic frontal view of the heart: 1, LMCA—left main coronary artery; 2, LAD—left anterior descending artery; 3, septal perforators of the LAD; 4, diagonal branch; 5, LCx—left circumflex artery; 6, OM—obtuse marginal branch of the LCx; 7, PDA—posterior descending artery; 8, RCA—right coronary artery; 9, SA nodal artery; 10, right ventricular (RV) branch; 11, acute marginal branches.

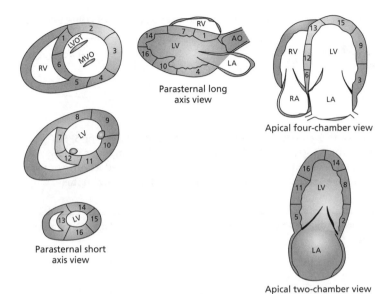

Parasternal long
axis view

Apical four-chamber view

Parasternal short
axis view

Apical two-chamber view

Figure A.10 Standard echocardiographic views: a 17-segment model for regional wall motion analysis, proposed by the American Society of Echocardiography. In the parasternal short axis view, the left ventricle (LV) is divided into three levels: basal, mid or papillary, and apical. The basal (segments 1–6) and the mid (segments 7–12) levels are subdivided into six segments each, while the distal level is divided into four segments. The true apex is segment 17. These 17 segments can be visualized in different planes, as depicted in the parasternal long axis, apical four-chamber axis, and apical two-chamber axis views. The anatomic nomenclature of each segment is depicted in the table below.

Segment level	Anteroseptal	Anterior	Lateral	Inferolateral	Inferior	Inferoseptal
Basal	1	2	3	4	5	6
Mid	7	8	9	10	11	12
Distal	13	14	15	–	16	13

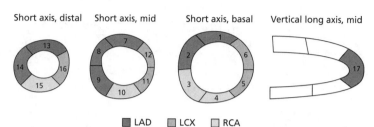

Figure A.11 Standard nuclear views: segmental division of the SPECT slices using the 17-segment model. The 17-segment scoring is as follows: 0 = normal; 1 = slight reduction in uptake; 2 = moderate reduction in uptake; 3 = severe reduction in uptake; 4 = absence of radioactive uptake:

Segment level	Anterior	Anteroseptal	Inferoseptal	Inferior	Inferolateral	Anterolateral
Basal	1	2	3	4	5	6
Mid	7	8	9	10	11	12
Distal	13	14	14	15	–	16

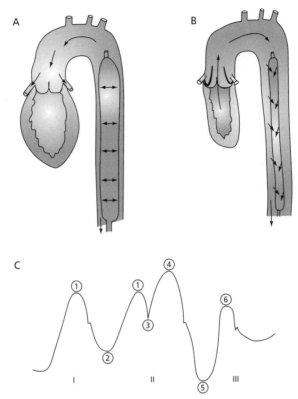

Figure A.12 The intraaortic balloon pump (IABP) is used in patients with refractory ischemia to stabilize them prior to a definitive revascularization. The major mode of action of the IAPB in unstable angina is improvement of diastolic coronary blood flow. Additionally, the mechanical action of inflation and deflation of the balloon causes afterload reduction and thus reduces myocardial wall stress. In diastole (A), the balloon is inflated, which raises the diastolic pressure and increases coronary artery perfusion. Just before and during systole (B), the balloon is quickly deflated, which decreases aortic pressure (decreases afterload) and thus promotes forward flow and facilitates cardiac output (adapted from Eugene Braunwald's *Atlas of Heart Diseases*). (C) Arterial waveforms during IABP assistance. Beats I and III are unassisted, and beat II is assisted with IABP in 2:1 mode: (1) is unassisted systole and (2) is unassisted aortic end-diastolic pressure; (3) is balloon inflation, resulting in diastolic augmentation (4) on the same beat, which improves coronary perfusion. This is followed by a lowered assisted aortic end-diastolic pressure (afterload) (5) due to balloon deflation, which decreases MVO_2 demand; while (6) is assisted systole.

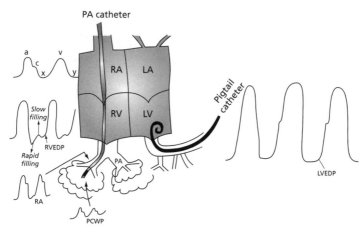

Figure A.13 Normal hemodynamic waveforms: a schematic drawing of normal pressure tracings obtained by a pulmonary artery catheter (the Swan–Ganz catheter) and a pigtail catheter in the left ventricle.

$$CO = \frac{O_2 \text{ consumption (nl/min)}}{AVO_2 \text{ difference (nlO}_2/100 \text{ ml blood)} \times 10}$$

AVO_2 difference $= 1.36 * Hb$ concentration*(Arterial sat − Mixed Venous sat)

O_2 consumption: estimated as 125 ml/min/m² or can be measured from a metabolic hood

$$CI = \frac{CO \text{ (ml/beat)}}{BSA \text{ (m}^2)}$$

$$SVR = \frac{\overline{MAP} - \overline{RA}}{CO} \text{ (Wood units)}$$

$$PVR = \frac{\overline{PAP} - \overline{PCWP}}{CO} \text{ (Wood units)}$$

Wood units*80 = Dynes*s*cm⁻⁵

Figure A.14 Basic hemodynamic calculations, utilizing the Fick Principle.

Index

Figures and Tables are indicated by *italic page numbers*, Boxes by **bold numbers**. Abbreviations: ACS = acute coronary syndrome; ECG = electrocardiography; MI = myocardial infarction; PCI = percutaneous coronary intervention; STEMI = ST-segment-elevation myocardial infarction; UA = unstable angina